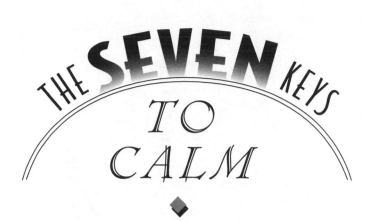

THE SEVEN KEYS TO CALM

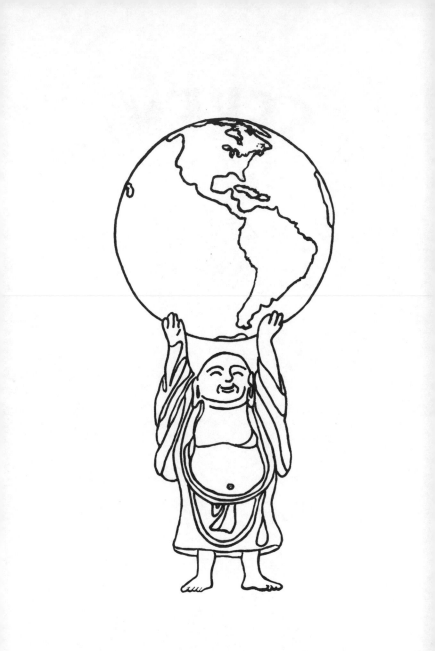

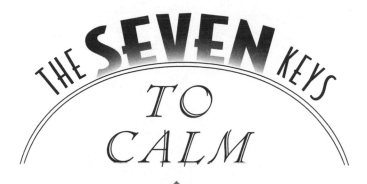

THE SEVEN KEYS TO CALM

ESSENTIAL STEPS FOR STAYING CALM UNDER ANY CIRCUMSTANCES

A. M. Matthews

POCKET BOOKS
New York   London   Toronto   Sydney   Tokyo   Singapore

POCKET BOOKS, a division of Simon & Schuster Inc.
1230 Avenue of the Americas, New York, NY 10020

ISBN: 0-671-00026-8

First Pocket Books hardcover printing September 1997

10 9 8 7 6 5 4 3 2 1

Illustration by Gary Uhl
Text design by Stanley S. Drate/Folio Graphics Co. Inc.

Printed in the U.S.A.

This book is dedicated to you
who found your way to it,
and to all the bodhisattvas
who help me find my own way.

CONTENTS

INTRODUCTION

ello. Welcome to this copy of *The Seven Keys to Calm*. If you've selected it from among the many, many titles on your bookstore or library shelves and have actually gotten so far as to read this introduction, I'll venture a guess about you:

Chances are you are a person who thinks of yourself as anything *but* calm. If asked to describe yourself, you'd set forth a portrayal of what is often termed the quintessential Type A personality— tense, impatient, preoccupied, on edge.

Plop you down in the middle of a traffic jam, or in a line at the motor vehicles department, and watch your toes tap and your fingers drum. Give you one frustration too many in the course of a day, and watch your temper flare, even though you keep telling yourself you won't let *that* happen anymore. Position you at an airport luggage carousel, and listen to that voice of doom in your head, assuring you that your bags are doubtless on their way to Quito, Ecuador, while you stand coatless in Cleveland.

If only, you often think to yourself, you could be like those enviable Type B's—calm, composed, sanguine, cheerful, approachable, more tolerant, and somehow more focused and centered. Then daily life would seem more of a blessing, and less of a chore.

You might offer up any number of theories as to why you are the type you are, and indeed they may be quite valid theories. Perhaps you come from a long line of histrionic ancestors who jump up and down, wring their hands, and invoke the gods when faced with little more than a hangnail. Perhaps you have been branded "cranky" or "high-strung" since earliest childhood and have developed some long-term anxious habits while living up to your designated role. Maybe you consider yourself especially sensitive to the chaotic world around you, counting yourself a victim of late-twentieth-century pervasive premillennial dread.

You probably consider your anxious attitude as fixed and permanent as a chunk of stone, and are dubious that anything can alter it. But Michelangelo—who knew more about the nature of stone than anyone—believed that each block of granite contained a glorious sculpture within. In order to get at the core and liberate it, what one needed to do was to chip away the excess on the outside.

That's what *The Seven Keys to Calm* is meant to accomplish. It is a program for removing obstacles to one's true inner nature—a nature that lies beneath all the entrenched anxious habits and which, in every one of us, embodies *an indestructible and infinitely replenishable core of calm just waiting to be accessed.*

A basic premise of *The Seven Keys to Calm* is that there are, in fact, no Type A people. There is only Type A *behavior* and *outlook.* No matter what your genetic and chemical makeup, your characterological bent, your family training, or your social and occupational milieu, you are inherently capable of returning to a home base of tranquillity and serenity, even in the face of great frustration or adversity. Indeed, just like Dorothy in Oz, you have had the power to go "home" all along. You just haven't known it.

Now you will.

Anxiety and calm coexist. They are like all dualities (up/down, empty/full, joy/sorrow): you simply cannot have one without the other. But we all have the power to *choose* calm. *The Seven Keys* consists of the information and techniques you will need in order to make that choice more and more often in the course of your daily existence.

Let me briefly summarize what you will encounter on your journey toward calm: The First Key, the Key of Clarity, places anxiety in a new context, so that we might control it rather than letting it control us. The Second Key, the Key of Compassion, offers a different way of dealing with those "troublesome" people we consider so provocative and stress-inducing. The Third Key, the Key of Crisis, discusses using the lessons of life's catastrophes to develop a new respect for our intrinsic powers and for our place in the world. The Fourth Key, the Key of Cycles, offers a rationale for celebrating, rather than fighting, the most fundamental law of the universe—which is change. The Fifth Key, the Key of Cessation, addresses coming to terms with the logical conclusion and ultimate challenge of that law of change—our own mortality. The Sixth Key, the Key of Connectedness, concerns rethinking the course of one's life from an altered perspective. The Seventh Key, the Key of Cultivation, is meant to string all the preceding keys together and to foster their use even when the temptation may be to revert to previous, habitual ways of being.

Lest you are wondering what, more specifically, you will be asked to undertake in the course of *The Seven Keys to Calm* program, I will tell you that its approach is one I've taken to calling *psychospiritual.* This may sound a bit lofty, but I don't mean it to. I simply found I had to offer something in response to the many times I have been asked whether I would define the techniques herein as psychological or spiritual—as if the two were mutually exclusive. If a term is required at all, I decided, only a hybrid could suffice. After all, where does psychology end and spirituality begin? That is like asking where, exactly, is the dividing line between mind and soul? Everywhere. Nowhere. Two miles up and take a left at the Dairy Queen.

Now if you find yourself bristling a bit at a word such as *soul*—perhaps wondering if, in order to undertake this program, you need to have unshakable belief in such things, fear not. Unshakable beliefs are not only not required, they are, in fact, a considerable nuisance. (It's hard to envision a bigger albatross around one's neck than an unrevisable notion.) On the contrary, all that's required is an open mind, a willingness to suspend *dis*belief and to consider some things in a new light.

This book grew out of my work as a psychotherapist (a job in which one is continually made witness to the devastating impact of anxiety on the quality of life) and out of my ever-widening interest in Eastern philosophies and religions, especially Buddhism. However, you won't find anything elaborately academic, esoteric, or otherworldly here. Indeed, if I have done my job, you will find the cornerstones of the program to be common sense and humor (which are, for my nickel, the two most powerful tools we have in our arsenal for transformation).

I do offer one caveat, however. Each of the

Seven Keys consists of information and suggested actions. If you absorb the information without attempting the actions, you will fall short of the results you desire. All you will have ingested are words, and words—potent as they may be—can only take you so far. As the philosopher Alan Watts said, "A menu is very useful, but it is no substitute for dinner."

It is recommended that after reading each key, you begin to put it into practice and incorporate it into your everyday life. If you prefer to plow ahead toward the book's conclusion before starting the program, that's certainly all right. But keep in mind that incorporating each key in turn will likely make for a smoother path.

Also, be aware that undertaking the suggested actions will probably feel strange at first. Not bad/strange, but exciting/strange, akin to moving into a new house and trying to grope your way around before you know where all the light switches are. Don't worry about it. This is how it's supposed to feel. The actions are designed as catalysts, not rigid rules and regulations. They will help you make the personal leaps of intuition necessary to attain a new level of calm. And ultimately, though they won't alter the world, they will profoundly alter your way of perceiving it.

Change works in myriad ways, more ways than we could ever quantify. Sometimes it works from the inside out. But often it works from the outside in—like Michelangelo chipping away at stone. This outside-in route is the path of the Seven Keys. All that's necessary is to try some things on for size. Then you will see how they come to fit.

Did you ever hear the story of the ugly troll who wanted to marry the kind and beautiful princess? First, he donned a mask and dressed as a handsome prince. He quickly realized that looking the part was not enough, however, so he began to act like a prince worthy of the princess. He was noble, gracious, and generous to all. It must have worked, for the princess married him, and they lived together happily. But one day she said to him, "I know you are wearing a mask. Take it off or I will leave you forever." Having no choice, her husband removed his mask. Underneath he was . . . a handsome, noble, and gracious prince.

The ancient Hindu scriptures, the *Upanishads,* contain the line: "As a man acts, so does he become. As a man's desire is, so is his destiny." The troll desired princeliness, and he found within himself the will to fulfill his desire. Accordingly, he was able to set aside whatever convictions he held about his own limitations.

Set aside your own such opinions for a while. Stop reminding yourself what you are not, and you will discover what you are . . . the soul of calm.

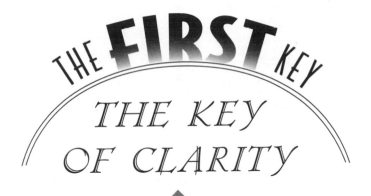

THE FIRST KEY

THE KEY OF CLARITY

◆

BE AWARE OF WHAT ANXIETY
IS, AND WHAT IT IS NOT.

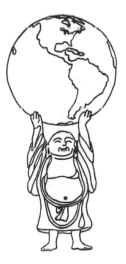

The wise man was asked, "How shall we escape the heat of the scorching flames?" He answered, "Go right into the middle of the fire."

—CHINESE APHORISM

To be happy is to become aware of oneself without fright.

—WALTER BENJAMIN

THE FIRST KEY TO CALM

*I*f you spend time with anyone in the five-year-old-and-under crowd, you may be intimately familiar with the Disney film *Bambi*—because little ones continually recruit grown-ups to sit with them during the scary parts. But if this ubiquitous video is not in your library, or currently logged into your short-term memory, allow me to describe a brief scene that illustrates a very useful lesson about anxiety:

A hunter enters the forest brandishing his rifle, and all of the animals race for cover. Three quails hide in the underbrush. The first quail repeatedly cries out in alarm as the hunter approaches. Her two friends warn her to be quiet. "Be calm," they whisper. "Don't get excited." But the first quail, in a panic, suggests that everyone fly. Her friends counter, "Whatever you do, don't fly." But, unable to tolerate another moment of such excruciating apprehension, the first quail propels herself upward. The inevitable *ka-blam* of gunfire follows.

We know someone will be roasting a quail for supper tonight.

What happened here? Why did two friends survive while another ended up an entrée? The lesson to be learned, in a nutshell: It's not anxiety per se that causes problems, but rather what one does with it. Learn to view anxiety with some objectivity and you can save yourself all manner of grief. Act rashly in hopes of getting rid of the feeling as quickly as possible and, as often as not, *ka-blam.*

The Scary Parts

All creatures experience anxiety—the quail, the whale, the hen, the fox, and, of course, the human being. It is part of the survival repertoire of every man and beast. Anxiety is brought into being by an expectation of possible danger and acts as a triggering mechanism, instigating hormonal and muscular responses that promote a state of alertness and a readiness to flee or to defend oneself if such behavior is required.

In many cases anxiety, whether instinctive or learned, is an appropriate response to a given set of circumstances. Should a cat come sniffing about a mouse hole, no one would call the mouse's emergent wariness a neurotic trait. And only a fool would suggest the restless rodent needed a healthy dose of "positive thinking" to counter its agitated mood.

Likewise, no one would fault a farmer whose anxiety compelled him to hurriedly ready his storm cellar when the weather forecast included tornadoes. Nor would one try to tempt him with a tranquilizer to take his mind off his troubles. Anxiety in this form—grounded in reality and focused on a tangible and imminent threat—should be afforded the healthy respect it deserves.

But anxiety, for all its evolutionary usefulness, can be problematical. For one thing, even when it is entirely appropriate to experience anxiety, one can overreact to it. Men or beasts who overreact and panic in the face of anxiety can hardly be expected to choose the wisest course of action. They might well expose themselves to unnecessary danger, either by selecting a course of action too impulsively or by becoming completely incapacitated, too overwhelmed by the feeling of anxiety to function.

For another thing, anxiety can sometimes manifest itself in inappropriate or extraneous ways, instigating a rehearsal for danger when, in fact, actual danger is *not* in the offing. This latter problem is endemic in our species.

In humankind, anxiety can take many insidious forms. It can also present abundant opportunities for reacting to it in a self-defeating manner. As you will see, clarity is the antidote for such self-defeat.

Junk Mail from the Mind

Like any other creature, of course, we humans sometimes experience specific, appropriate anxiety that warns us of genuine prospective peril. We hear a smoke alarm go off or see a toddler venture too close to a beehive, and we gear up for urgent action.

But let's be honest. We also tend to conjure up ingenious variations on this presumption-of-peril theme. For we humans tend to define *peril* broadly—that is, as anything that threatens to disrupt circumstances with which we have grown comfortable, or that even threatens to disrupt a vision of the future as we would *like* it to unfold.

For example, have you ever felt anxious about certain events occurring even though you had no objective information whatsoever that they would occur at all? (As in "I'm taking a vacation to Mexico in two weeks. I hope my plane doesn't crash. I hope it doesn't rain once I get there. I hope I don't come down with Montezuma's revenge.")

Have you ever dreaded performing your usual chores because something *un*usual—and, by your definition of *unusual,* awful—might happen? (As in "I have to get my car inspected. What if it takes forever and I'm too late to pick up the kids? What if that odd little clunk in the engine turns out to be some huge problem? What if I need a whole new transmission? How much is all this going to cost me?")

Have you ever felt you are mentally twisting yourself into a pretzel, desperately trying to will a particular situation (say a job interview or a medical exam) to turn out in a very particular way? Or, more impossible yet, trying to will everything in a current situation to stay exactly the way it is forevermore? And have you ever felt certain something bad was going to happen . . . you just weren't quite sure what?

If you've answered affirmatively, it's not because you're crazy, or stupid. In fact, it's because you're so smart. Your human brain is capable of the higher functions of imagining, fantasizing, calculating, and prognosticating. It is capable of contemplating not only the immediate future, but long-term probabilities and possibilities.

Certainly the human brain is a wondrous, awe-inspiring thing, with many laudable accomplishments to its credit (mathematics, music, chemistry, astronomy . . . *ad infinitum*). But when it comes to anxiety, the forever-forward-thinking human brain is wont to run amok. For along with the imperative anxiety-provoking communications it sends us ("Smoke alarm beeping: Check it out!" "Bees buzzing around your kid. Take note!"), it also sends us a massive amount of junk mail.

Junk mail from your mind is not unlike the junk

mail in your mailbox. It is full of messages that activate a continual stream of wishes and fears.

The junk mail in your mailbox may tell you life would be more complete if only you took a cruise to the Bahamas, joined a health club, or purchased, say, a goose down comforter, a new set of power tools, or a thigh-and-buttock toner. It might also urge you to consider a new credit card with which to purchase this assortment, and perhaps a credit card protection policy in case someone attempts to obtain all these goodies for himself at your expense.

Now this may all seem like so much superfluous stuff and nonsense—which indeed it is—but consider for a moment how often one's mind hums similar refrains. "Got to get some more of this," croons the mind. "You can never have too much of that." And: "Now that you've got it, you'd better make sure you keep it. What would you do if you lost it?"

This continual craving for ways to alter the course of our lives, ostensibly for the better, and desire to exert control (especially over what is uncontrollable) make us endlessly anxious. Yet the mind can be so ingenious and so relentless that we grow completely habituated to its assiduous, insatiable desires, imagining that the anxious life they bid us to lead is the only life there is.

And so we become junk mail junkies. But we need not be.

A New Approach

As diverted as you may be by the junk mail in your mailbox, you would hardly consider taking action on every piece of it that came your way. For the most part, you probably sort through it quickly, perhaps getting a good chuckle out of some of it. Then you put aside what's not really relevant to your circumstances or needs (very likely most, if not all, of it).

Yet we very often feel compelled to react strongly to the mind's little missives. Because, hey, after all, it's our magnificent mind talking, right? Our constant companion. Our ever vigilant arbiter of reality. So we must need to do *something* when the mind serves up an anxious thought. But what should we do?

Imagine, for example, rolling around in bed trying to get to sleep when the mind decides to send a message that says, more or less, "Ahem, remember that article you read in the paper yesterday that said the IRS is planning more tax audits this year. Were you really entitled to all those deductions?" Or "Yo there, trying to get to sleep, are you? Well, have you taken some time today to think about whether or not you're really going to have enough money for retirement?" Or "Noticed those extra hairs on your hairbrush tonight. Doesn't baldness run in your family?" Now we can hardly indulge in a quintessential fight or flight response in reaction to such thoughts. There's nowhere to run and there's no one to fight with.

But we don't much care for being stuck with the way the thoughts make us feel. We experience the feelings as burdensome, irritating, and altogether unpleasant. We want to obliterate them at any cost. We want to take action.

So maybe we do attempt to fight—with ourselves. We try to dispute all the scary scenarios our mind has conjured up. (Though the resourceful mind just comes up with new, scarier ones.) And maybe we do try to run—jumping out of bed to down a Xanax or Valium to try to make our feelings go away. (Though now we'll be anxious about when to take our next pill, and anxious that the doctor may not renew our prescription since we're taking them a little more often than recommended.)

Or maybe we just stew and mull, fret and worry, until the worry becomes an end in itself. Or maybe we store the anxiety in our bodies, generating everything from heartburn to headaches to far more serious conditions.

Now let me suggest an alternative. One that you may have never considered. What if, instead of taking these kinds of habitual actions in response to anxiety, we were able to *just look* at our anxiety dispassionately and sort through it with a detached, objective eye before deciding what action to take—if any at all? That is where the Key of Clarity comes in.

Understanding the Key of Clarity

The Key of Clarity is about developing a discriminating awareness where anxiety is concerned. It states: *Be aware of what anxiety is and what it is not.*

So what is anxiety? It is a *message* from the mind

that warns that danger lurks and a *feeling* of wanting to respond to that message.

What is anxiety not? It is *not our master, but our servant.* So long as we refuse to give it absolute power over us, it can help rather than harm us.

When we empower anxiety we rush frantically to answer its call and quell its siren song. Even when the danger is a very tangible one, the consequences of such undiscerning haste are often negative. They can range from the embarrassing (imagine calling for the fire department when your beeping smoke alarm is signaling nothing other than a low battery) to the injurious (imagine waving your arms about excitedly to fend off a bee, and thus bringing about the very sting you dread) to the terminal (remember the quail who felt she *had* to fly rather than wait out the hunter in silence).

When the mind's "red alert" is heeded and the peril we dread is, in fact, only an imagined one, equally disastrous consequences can ensue. We hardly need to be further convinced of the ill effects of stress on health. Many believe that chronic anxiety can, quite literally, affect the length of our lives. And it undeniably affects the day-to-day *quality* of our lives. In a sorry paradox, our minds' continual jabbering about potential "threats" to our equanimity makes that very equanimity impossible to achieve. It separates us from the good life we say we want to live.

Remember, however, the mind is persistently yakety-yakking. One might say that is its job. Like a talk-show host bucking for ratings, it is deeply determined to make a big deal out of something, even if that something turns out to be nothing much in the end.

Trying to prevent the mind from manufacturing anxious thoughts is futile. Nabisco would sooner stop manufacturing saltines. But prevention of thoughts *isn't* necessary or desirable. What's needed is an ability to pause, however briefly, *when the thought first registers* and evaluate the stimulus that engendered it in the first place. With even a millisecond of rational evaluation, we can detach from our anxiety and assess whether or not a danger is real. If it is real, we will know, in our objectivity, how best to act. If it isn't real, we can discard the anxious thought like a piece of unwanted junk mail.

To pause is everything. For in the gap of detached scrutiny that the pause creates, anxiety finally loosens its grip on us. In that gap lies the serenity and tranquillity we find so elusive.

But just how does one pause? To borrow an old vaudeville line, it's the same way one gets to Carnegie Hall: practice, practice, practice.

The Key of Clarity in Action

Anxiety, you'll recall, always entails a warning. And a warning, by definition, is an anticipation of something that might happen. So anxiety is about what *might* happen as opposed to what *is* happening. When we are slaves to anxiety, we're constantly living in the realm of "might," which is to say, in the future. To end this enslavement we must actively practice living in the land of "is," which is to say, in the moment.

Now you may protest: "But I already live in the moment." Do you? In a well-known Zen tale, a disciple asks a master what he understands to be the secret of life. The master replies, "When I eat, I eat. When I sleep, I sleep." How many of us can say the same?

When we eat we think about what we're going to eat next, and calculate how many fat grams we're consuming, and worry how we're going to look in a bathing suit, and think of dozens of other scenarios that have nothing at all to do with the food in front of us or the experience of eating it. When we sleep, we toss and turn and wake with a start at four A.M., realizing that even in "sleep" we've been pondering the potential dangers and difficulties in our lives. When we're at work, we think of being home. And when we're home, we think of being at work. We're simply never where we are.

This mind-set, however, can be gradually altered.

To reconnect to the moment and defuse anxiety's power over us, we can begin by choosing to deliberately focus on one thing—and only one thing—that is happening now.

For ten minutes every day, try undertaking a single activity and concentrating fully on *it*. For example, when you eat, *eat*. Commit a fraction of each day to, say, eating a bowl of soup with full attentiveness. Don't talk while you eat it, and don't read or watch TV. Don't worry about how much sodium is in the soup. Don't wish for a new bowl to eat it in. Don't judge the soup or rate it. Just taste it, smell it, experience its texture and temperature. If

(I should say *when*) your mind wanders, gently
bring it back to the activity at hand.

You can apply this attentiveness practice to virtually anything. Take a bath with attentiveness.
Peel potatoes. Scrub some pots. Or just place a
flower on your desk and, from time to time, look
at it with attentiveness. Become as resourceful in
finding things to pay full attention to in the moment as you are in finding things to obsess on
which may or may not happen in the future. (And
if you need a personal instructor, just observe a
very young child devoting attention to any commonplace activity or object, for very young children
are naturally awestruck by whatever is engaging
them.)

Bringing attentiveness to commonplace experiences creates an opportunity for the mind to settle
down and achieve clarity. But, I warn you, this
seemingly simple practice also creates powerful
challenges and can be highly frustrating at first. Because among the things you will see clearly, probably for the first time, is how frantically your mind
tries to flee from the present moment, often using
anxiety as its chief means of transportation.

It is inevitable that anxious thoughts will interject themselves into your attentiveness practice. But it can't be emphasized strongly enough *that this does not mean you are doing anything wrong.* On the contrary. Roll out the welcome mat for those anxious thoughts! By showing up right now, they are providing you, at long last, with a means for managing them.

Who's the Boss?

So when you're minding your own business, attempting to polish the silver or repot a plant attentively, and your mind sends you nagging, anxious little missives, don't try to banish them. It's like telling yourself not to think of purple porpoises. Inevitably, purple porpoises will soon be all you're thinking about.

Don't struggle against the thoughts either. For like an insect caught in a Venus flytrap, the more you struggle, the more tightly you are encased.

Don't try to replace a thought with its opposite. Remember Ralph Kramden, the volatile *Honeymooners* character who tried to convince himself he was not upset by insisting, through clenched teeth and locked jaw, "Pins and needles, needles and pins, a happy man is a man who grins." He was not fooling anyone, of course, least of all himself. And neither will you.

Above all, try not to get all involved with the thoughts and cling to them—as is our entrenched habit—for dear life.

Without judgment, and without labeling the thoughts "good" or "bad," just notice them. Watch their fleeting nature. Bear them in mind momentarily, acknowledge them, and then bring your attention back to your chosen focused activity.

Now, your anxious thoughts are not used to being treated in this fashion. They will likely revisit you in short order, tugging at the sleeve of your consciousness, whining, "Hey, didn't you hear what I said?" You may give them a mental smile and nod (perhaps beginning to see traces of humor in their mischievous persistence). But in once again turning your attention to the *now,* you are, in effect, reminding your anxious thoughts that even though they may keep coming back, they cannot stick around.

Now you are actually beginning to show who's in charge around here. And, lo and behold, it's not your thoughts after all. It's something larger, purer, and far more enduring. It's Awareness with a capital A.

It's as if thoughts are the many brushstrokes that make up a painting. Beneath and behind the brushstrokes and the picture they comprise, however, is a canvas. The canvas holds or "houses" the painting. But the canvas itself doesn't alter because of what's imposed on its surface. Fundamentally, it is immutable. If you could peer beneath the overlay of paint, or gently wash it away with solvent, you would see it in its pure state—clear and spacious. Simply to realize that the canvas underlies the painting at all times is to take the first step toward liberation from anxiety's tyranny.

The Power of Awareness

Henry Miller wrote, "The aim of life is to live, and to live means to be aware, joyously, drunkenly, serenely, divinely aware." Virtually everyone who studies the workings of the mind—from experimental psychologists to psychoanalysts to spiritual philosophers—is convinced of the beneficial effects of cultivating awareness.

Psychologists will attest that if we process an emotion through the brain's neocortex (which is the physiological description of the awareness process), the odds of handling it appropriately vastly improve. Psychoanalysts will point out that the trademark of the mentally fit is the ability to let an impulse arise and pass away, briefly holding it in awareness without acting on it imprudently. Buddhists will tell you that generating the sort of awareness that comes from focused attention is the first step toward attaining *nirvana*—the state of bliss brought about by the absence of continual longings and desires. These are all different ways of conceptualizing the same truth, namely, that awareness ultimately can break any destructive emotional cycle.

None of this goes to disparage emotions and emotional thoughts themselves, which give life so much of its rich texture. It is only to say that we ought to conceptualize them differently. We should honor them, but we must not blindly worship them to the exclusion of all else. And to truly honor thoughts and feelings we need to look at them without prejudice or preconception.

Think of the manifestations of your hustling,

bustling, ever-chatting mind as part of your sensory array. You don't believe, nor do you instantly react to, everything you see or hear—at least not without further investigation. And though at first it may seem strange to contemplate, you can't believe everything you think either.

Of Two Minds

In a way, it is as if each of us has two minds. There is, of course, the perennially Busy Mind, doing its valuable workaday chores, but also continually fussing like a mother duck over her ducklings. But then there is the Calm Mind, stable and steadfast. Unflappable. It is, as the Indian teacher and philosopher Krishnamurti so eloquently put it, "a mind that is not distracted by its own thought."

The Busy Mind is to brushstrokes as the Calm Mind is to the canvas beneath them. Become acquainted with the Calm Mind *(which you already possess, whoever you are)* for even a few minutes at a time, and cumulative benefits will rapidly reveal themselves.

Your inappropriate anxieties will lose their hold on you, as you begin to see that reacting to them is merely a habit that can be broken. Even when faced with a genuine cause for anxiety, you will be able to conduct yourself all the more wisely for having learned that you can create some vital distance between yourself and any given situation. Now, instead of panicking, you will be an eye of calm in the storm of anxiety. Instead of overanalyzing a problem and tearing it apart only to grow increasingly frustrated, you will find that solutions will begin to present themselves to you more quickly and intuitively.

In the bargain, you will begin to "lighten up," take yourself less seriously, and laugh at many more things than you ever did before, especially yourself. In fact, when the Chicken Littles of anxiety come clucking at all hours, insisting that the sky is falling, you may find yourself responding with a knowing grin instead of running for cover.

Who Says So?

In the initial weeks, the going may be slow. Replacing an ingrained habit with a new one always involves the proverbial two steps forward, one step back. But undertaking attentiveness practice for a little while each day is actually the fastest route to removing the obstacles that stand between you and your naturally Calm Mind.

I know you'd like me to prove it. And, in fact, I could tell you that for over five millennia, saints, mystics, and shamans (all of them innate "psychologists") of every tradition have conducted what are, for all intents and purposes, experiments verifying the dramatic effects that practicing "now-focused" attention can have on day-to-day disposition. Though they may call the source of peacefulness and equanimity they access by different names (a Buddhist may say *the Buddha nature,* a Christian *the Holy Spirit,* a Sufi *the Hidden Essence,* a Hindu *the Atman,* and so forth), their insights all attest to its universality. The naturally Calm Mind is no less a part of any one of us than it is of them. They've just put the time and effort into looking for it.

But I won't belabor this issue, because the real point here is that, finally, no one can really prove any of this to you but yourself. Do your own experiment: Try a few minutes of attentiveness to a sole activity each day for, say, three weeks. Then stop for a week. (Stopping will be a cakewalk, because the tug of old habits and the Busy Mind that enforces them will have been nagging you to stop this "foolishness" anyway.) Now observe yourself at the end of your week off and notice the differences in the way you conduct yourself.

How does your stress level differ? How much time are you spending ruminating about things you cannot change? How are you reacting in the face of life's ups and downs? How do you feel about yourself? And how are you treating other people? The answers should speak for themselves, but if they are not resoundingly clear, then ask those people who are close to you if they have noticed any changes. You may be surprised how differently others perceive you depending on whether or not you are accessing your Calm Mind.

*T*his, by the way, brings us to the Second Key to Calm, which focuses on our dealings with one another—because, unlike monks and mystics who may nourish their Calm Mind in the privacy of a monastery or a sacred cave, you will be cultivating yours in the real world. *Real* is a relative term, of course, but what I mean is the world of spouses, children, in-laws, bosses and subordinates, friends and neighbors.

Ours is the world of people who neglect to turn off their car alarms, who bring eighteen items to the express line of the supermarket, and who make telemarketing phone calls to you just as you are sitting down to dinner. If you sometimes feel all of them seem to exist to make your life more complicated and to goad you into losing your Calm Mind rather than using it, please read on.

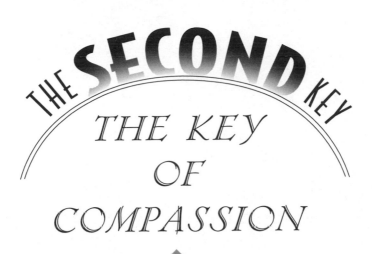

THE SECOND KEY

THE KEY
OF
COMPASSION

◆

SUBSTITUTE COMPASSION
FOR CONTROL.

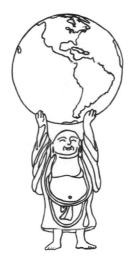

Compassionate generosity . . . is the
practice of letting go.

—JACK KORNFIELD

Not expecting anything, we do not get
impatient.

—CHOGYAM TRUNGPA

THE SECOND KEY TO CALM

Shortly after my son turned two, the universe saw fit to offer me a little lesson in how my anxious Busy Mind likes to butt into everyone else's business. One afternoon, Skyler was happily playing with his Thomas the Tank Engine train set. All of a sudden he started dismantling his track and placing pieces of it onto the lap of a large armchair in the living room. Excitedly running back and forth from his train table to the chair, he then piled several of his trains and other toy railway accoutrements atop the heap of track segments. Then, he added several stuffed animals to the pile. Next, some wooden blocks. Next, some odds and ends from his toy chest. All the while, he giggled with purposeful glee.

I sat on the sofa watching, first with mild curiosity, then with a suspiciously widening agenda. What was he attempting, I wondered? What was his plan? He seemed so definitive about what he was doing. Was he constructing a piece of artwork? A sculpture of some sort? Something that would assure me he was destined for the Harvard track? I was sure all this fevered and focused activity was some sort of testament to my child's extraordinary abilities—but in what way?

"Honey," I asked him anxiously, "what are you making?"

"Mama," he answered, quite pleased with himself, "I'm making a mess."

Had he been a few years older he might have added, "Gee, Mom, how can you be so dense?"

*H*ow *could* I be so dense? Easy. Like anyone consumed with genuine love for another, I fell into one of the Busy Mind's most common traps. Instead of just enjoying and appreciating my son's revels, and letting him make his own mess, I wanted to anticipate the outcome of what he was doing. I wanted him to make me proud. I wanted him to prove that my fantasies about him were justified. I wanted, in a literal sense, to impose my constructs on his.

How easy it is to get anxious on behalf of people we love. We want them to be happy, of course. But we rarely question that we should be the ones who decide what constitutes their happiness. We want them to conform to our wishes for them, and on the one hand *expect* them to. On the other hand, we live in fear that they'll be swayed by some alternate agenda.

We worry almost ceaselessly in this fashion about our children, about our spouses, about our aging parents, and about our friends. Ironically, the more certain we are about how all of them should conduct their lives, the more anxious, angry, and frustrated we feel. It's a burden being right all the time—and we have little doubt we *are* right.

Of course, the Busy Mind isn't satisfied with knowing what's best only when it comes to people we care for. It also insists that it knows best about people we don't care for so much. And about people we don't even know.

Other People, Other Plans

Think, for a moment, of all the people with whom you come into contact in the course of a day whose not-so-exemplary behavior you fervently wish you could alter:

- the co-worker who always sucks up to the boss
- the boss who prefers a suck-up to someone of real talents—such as yourself
- the annoying neighbor whose rhododendrons keep encroaching on your turf
- the guy who sat next to you on the train this morning and rattled his newspaper in your face for the whole ride
- the insurance salesman who kept trying to sell you a whole-life policy when you only wanted term
- that weather forecaster who actually seems to gloat when there's a blizzard because it means *he* was right

- the CEO of the computer company you hold stock in who stood idly by as share prices plummeted
- that lady in the Volvo who sped up as you were trying to pass

You believe the world would be a better place (and your life a better life) if only you could straighten them out about a few things. And for all practical purposes, "practical" at least from your perspective, you may have some valid ideas. But the very intensity of your belief in your "rightness" and their "wrongness" causes you all manner of stress.

How many of these people can get under your skin? How many of them can disrupt the tenor of your day and alter your mood dramatically? How many of them can get you to forfeit your equanimity, causing you to seethe silently or pop off publicly? Most likely your answer is all of them—at least some of the time.

But the truth is, as long as you are emotionally invested in wishing to control others, you empower those others to wreak havoc with your state of mind, causing you a world of harm. Invest in com-

passion as an alternative, and you do everyone a
world of good, including—and especially—yourself. For when you substitute compassion for control, you will soon see that *the only person who can
force you to renounce your Calm Mind is you.*

This is not to say that other people are not going
to attempt to thwart your intentions from time to
time. They will, naturally enough, because they
have intentions and agendas of their own, which
have to do with establishing *their* territory and fos-
tering *their* security. But rather than thinking of
people whose plans are at cross-purposes with our
own as hindrances, we can elect to think of them
as our teachers. Because it is only with their assistance, unwitting though it may be, that we can
learn to utilize the Second Key to Calm.

Understanding the Key of Compassion

The Key of Compassion states: *Substitute compassion for control.* But just what is compassion?

Most of us equate the concept with words such
as *kindness, generosity,* and *empathy*—all of which
are, indeed, its makings. But when it is absolutely
genuine, compassion must also encompass the

concepts of *universality* and *impartiality*. True compassion is freely given to all. What's more, it is never undertaken with the idea of self-aggrandizement. (Meaning, one doesn't do it merely in order to think, "Gee, what a swell person I am.")

Buddhist imagery portrays compassion by depicting a moon shining in the sky and reflecting in a hundred bowls of water. The moon shines on all the bowls, offering its light indiscriminately, and without reservation. Moreover, it neither asks nor expects anything in return. It just shines peacefully on.

Compassion has been defined by many philosophers as a yardstick of grace. It is also a gauge of calm. For it enables us to contain the rampant anxiety that grows out of continually angling to promote our agendas over everyone else's.

Much of our anxiety grows out of the belief that we are completely separate and set apart from everyone else, which leads to ongoing efforts in subtle (or not-so-subtle) one-upmanship. Because if everyone is separate, some must be "superior" to others, mustn't they? Calm, however, supplants anxiety when we begin with the assumption that life is an ensemble production, in which we all costar.

In modern Western society, we are typically trained to prize individuality above all, and the assertion that all of us are, in fact, parts of a consummate whole may seem at first like so much ethereal gobbledygook. But folk song lyrics and New Age niceties notwithstanding, the objective reality is that all humans—and indeed all earthly creatures—are not just metaphorically but actually, verifiably related.

Eons ago, the elements that comprise each one of us (the hydrogen, oxygen, iron, nitrogen, and carbon that are the constituents of life) were scattered across the galaxy in a series of supernova explosions. We were all born of the stars and, as renowned astronomer Allan Sandage has put it, we were once "all together in the same nebula."

None other than Albert Einstein has made eloquent assertions of our ultimate interconnectedness. "A human being is part of a whole," he said, "called by us the 'Universe,' a part limited in time and space. He experiences himself, his thoughts and feelings, as something separated—a kind of optical delusion of his consciousness." The revered scientist went on to describe this delusion as "a kind of prison for us, restricting us to our personal desires and to affection for a few persons nearest us."

Finding one's way out of this prison begins with the completely rational recognition that although each of us is a unique being, we are all interdependent on one another. The ultimate jailbreak occurs when we can actually imagine what it feels like to assess the world from another being's point of view. The application of a dose of empathic universal compassion allows us to gain all-important, calming awareness in situations that formerly made us react angrily, anxiously, or fearfully.

For example, in my psychotherapy practice I worked with a woman, whom I'll call Caroline, who had an acute dislike of insects, especially spiders. As fate would have it, spiders proliferated in the small vacation house she and her husband purchased in the country. Whenever she saw one, she would scream bloody murder, jump up and down, and demand that her husband "do something with it." Her husband would gently coax the poor arachnid onto a piece of paper and escort it out of doors, shaking his head all the while. Afterward, Caroline said, she "felt like a jerk."

Try as we might to get to the bottom of Caroline's spider anxiety, we could unearth no past traumatic incident involving a spider. Nor did she believe that spiders symbolized any other particular menace for which they were playing psychic surrogates. She just thought they were "disgusting and gross, all creepy-crawly." Finally, I asked her if she ever thought to look at what happened from the spider's perspective: there's a spider hanging out in your living room, minding his own business, when in walks this enormous person who starts pointing, jumping up and down, and shrieking at the top of her lungs. What do you think *he* thinks, I asked her.

"Well, if you put it that way," said Caroline, "probably, 'Yikes, look at that huge screaming thing! What does she want from my life?'"

Probably that, or something very much like it.

From then on, bit by bit, Caroline calmed down about spiders. She figured out that the only threat being posed to her came from inside her. She learned to walk a compassionate mile in the spider's shoes—all eight of them—and realized that in the grand scheme of things, she and the spider were on the same page. They both wanted to hang out around the house, tending to their own affairs, in peace.

The Key of Compassion in Action

Granted, it's not always easy to see things from someone else's point of view and to peacefully co-exist as a result. It's hard enough to do with a spider, and infinitely more challenging with, say, your teenage daughter.

In attempting to substitute compassion for control we will come up against many pitfalls. It's difficult even to conceive of attaining the calm that grows from universal compassion when we're so preoccupied with a few central characters in our lives, anxiously obsessing on how we can "help" them.

But not all kinds of selective "help" are truly compassionate. And many kinds of help aren't even really helpful.

Is it helpful to aid an alcoholic in drinking secretly? Obviously not. Is it helpful to do all a child's homework for him? Just as obviously, that would be to the child's disadvantage. Is it helpful to try to protect a loved one so she never has to face the harsh realities of life? Here things get a little fuzzy. We'd very much like to. In fact, we are often tormented by anxiety because we fear we will not be able to pull off such a monumental feat. But suppose we *could* pull it off?

In laboratory experiments involving cats, it was noted that many mother cats would allow their kittens to chase mice but would intervene if they chased rats. Tested apart from their mothers, the kittens proved quite able to take on the rats themselves. If their mothers had hung around indefinitely, one doubts the kittens would ever have had their chance to prove themselves.

We need to allow those we love opportunities to test their own abilities. Yes, we can help nurture their strengths and yes, we can warn them against recklessness. We can *influence* them, but really we can't control what happens to them, or how they respond to what happens. Even if we could, it would not serve them. Nor would it serve us in the long run. Think about it: Do you really want the responsibility of being your brother's—or lover's or best friend's—keeper? What a Busy Mind you would have then!

To begin to put the Key of Compassion into action, try asking yourself, when you catch yourself feverishly, almost painfully absorbed in the logistics of how you are going to "help" a loved one: Do you want to *assist* or to *prevail?* Are you motivated out of respect for the person's point of view or are you invested in attaining something for yourself (perhaps something as subtle as a feeling of self-satisfaction)? If control is your driving force, resist the temptation to intervene. If you can honestly offer no-strings-attached assistance while honoring the other's perspective, do so. You will be able both to make yourself useful and to keep yourself calm, *because you won't have your ego all tied up in the outcome of things.*

Moreover, try not to orchestrate "help" on a grand—and grandiose—scale. You will drive yourself mad trying to "fix" everything for everyone, and could well end up making things worse by attempting to take on too much.

Bear in mind the words of William Blake, who wisely cautioned, "He who would do good to another must do it in Minute Particulars." And if you have trouble learning to limit your help to Minute Particulars where your closest loved ones are concerned, don't worry. The universe has generously provided each of us with a limitless number of ideal people to practice on: absolute strangers.

Small Good Things

Many religious philosophies and ethical systems counsel their followers to undertake at least one small, arbitrary act of kindness in the course of each day. In Judaism, the worthy deed is called a *mitzvah;* in Boy Scouting it's simply a "good turn." But whatever it's called, the task is the same: to selflessly assist one person, even if that person is utterly unknown to you, in precisely the way he or she needs to be assisted at that moment.

This doesn't mean writing strangers into your will, cosigning their mortgage, or inviting them to spend a few weeks at your time share condo. It simply means being alert to the little predicaments in which people find themselves and making things a little easier or pleasanter for them as they cope with whatever is theirs to cope with.

What's the goal here? Not to pry piously into

other people's affairs. Not to grandiosely attempt to affect sweeping changes in the course of history. Not to preen or to remind other people what truly nice individuals we are. The goal is to train ourselves in compassion. As we do so, we also train ourselves to calm down.

Numerous ways to help people will present themselves when you start looking. (The traveler who needs directions, the newcomer who could use a friendly word, the eight-year-old or the eighty-year-old who just needs to have his jokes laughed at.) The point is *the very act of looking will help you attain and maintain calm* because you will be more attuned to the moment and to what surrounds you, and less preoccupied with your Busy Mind's anxious desires and dreads.

Cultivating an attitude of alertness to the kinds of struggles everyone shares lets you understand that you have by no means cornered the market on problems and worries. Realizing that we are all in it together makes your own anxieties seem far less central, and far less oppressive.

Once again, keep your aspirations modest and focus on what will gratify the person you are assisting, as opposed to your ego. It takes a while to get the knack of performing selflessly in Minute Particulars, because the Busy Mind is so habitually insistent that we should *do something* in order to *get something*.

I recall many years ago when I was first introduced to the idea of *karma,* the spiritual principle of eternally resonating causes and effects that impact destiny (a kind of cosmic domino theory in which good begets good and harm begets more harm). At the time I erroneously understood karma to signify short-term deals one makes with the cosmos in which one gets back precisely and literally what one gives out—and fast. One day I entered a New York City taxicab and was presented with what I saw to be an opportunity to instantly improve my personal karma. A previous passenger had dropped her checkbook on the floor. On reaching my office, I was able to track the woman down and happily offer to return it, magnanimously refusing any offer of monetary reward.

Aha, I thought to myself. I have made a deposit in my karmic bank account. Now the next time I lose something it will come right back to me. My hopes were high. And in short order, several things

I valued or depended on were indeed lost. My driver's license, a set of keys, and a favorite earring all vanished.

Alas, they were never to be seen by me again.

I consulted a friend of mine, a meditation instructor more fully acquainted than I with such matters. "What gives?" I asked. To which he replied that the purpose of daily *mitzvahs* was not to hedge against a rainy day, but to reaffirm the unity of all living things.

In turn, I humbly remind you: Helping a proverbial little old lady across the street is fine (provided she actually wants to cross the street). But once you help her across, don't stand by the side of the road congratulating yourself and anxiously awaiting immediate reciprocity from the universe. You might get splattered by a passing truck. Your worthy deed will be a deposit in your karmic bank account, all right. However, its yield will most likely not be a tangible bonus. Instead, it will be the psychic repose that comes from a Calm Mind that is not self-absorbed and does not create, or dwell on, barriers between the self and others.

Separated at Birth

Sigmund Freud wrote, "The act of birth is the first experience of anxiety," adding that birth anxiety was a "prototype," or model, of later anxieties to come. Many other psychologists agree that the separation of a child from the perfectly nurturing "oneness" of the womb underlies many of our more vague and extraneous anxieties. At the root of the Busy Mind's seemingly limitless desires there is the primal craving to feel utterly, wombishly safe and have all needs met before they are even experienced as needs. Alongside the craving there is the primal dread that this will never happen, that paradise is truly lost.

The catch is that so long as we look at the world from an egocentric point of view, imagining that "I" am in here and "everyone else" is out there, we can never regain what was lost, we can never be free of separation anxiety and all the self-torment it entails.

So, what to do? Einstein, remember, called separateness a delusion. It's a delusion, however, that is hard to give up on. In our culture, we cling to the notion that we're on our own, even as we ceaselessly try to get around it by, for example, searching for the perfect relationship we imagine will allow us to transcend our isolation. Then we find out our latest object of infatuation is unable to meet our needs perfectly and magically (and is unwilling to be controlled) and we grow disappointed, only to search for the next idealized "savior." Meanwhile, we neglect the solution staring straight at us: to feel calm and whole, we need to remember we are already part of a whole.

Alas, this solution is easier to embrace intellectually than emotionally. In other words, as much as we think we understand it, we find it difficult to put into practice. That is because, as Carl Jung put it, the egocentric consciousness "hypnotizes itself and therefore cannot be argued with."

All right, so we can't argue with it. We can still beat it at its own game. For a few weeks, no matter what you "believe" or "don't believe" or "think you believe," just *act as if you knew* that all of us were truly related, truly interdependent on each other. Assume that, as the late physician and essayist Lewis Thomas speculated, consciousness is a "generalized mechanism shared round not only among ourselves but with all the other conjoined things of the biosphere."

Then behave accordingly. Examine your motives. Don't attempt to get other people to fulfill your agenda. Make yourself useful. Assist but don't intervene. And cultivate what one Tibetan spiritual leader called "a sense of friendliness to everything." Then see what happens.

You will see that what you have created is compassion—universal, objective, and selfless. And *you will experience this compassion as one of the best antitoxins for your anxiety.*

Now you are ready to move on to yet another.

*T*he Key of Compassion teaches us that we cannot control others. In the next key this principle is expanded. The Key of Crisis is about surrendering the illusion that we can—and should—always control the events that befall us.

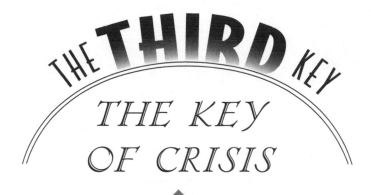

THE THIRD KEY

THE KEY OF CRISIS

◆

VIEW EACH CRISIS AS A CRASH
COURSE IN CALM.

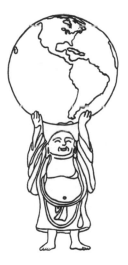

My foot slips on a narrow ledge: in that split second, as needles of fear pierce heart and temples, eternity intersects with present time.

—PETER MATTHIESSEN

Simplicity is action without idea. And that is what we do in crisis.

—KRISHNAMURTI

[Crisis] is the exquisite agony which a man might not want to experience again—yet would not for the world have missed.

—RICHARD NIXON

THE THIRD KEY TO CALM

*I*n a memoir, David Livingstone, the nine-
teenth-century African explorer who set out to find
the source of the Nile, recounted a vivid tale of
being caught by a lion and squeezed in its jaws.
He survived only because he was saved, at the last
possible moment, by a friend's marksmanship and
some extraordinary luck. Livingstone recalled the
episode in great detail. And he claimed he experienced, at the very moment he was in gravest danger of being gummed into oblivion, an astounding
sensation of *pure calm*.

Was his attitude in the face of immediate crisis an anomaly—perhaps because he was, by nature, a daring and adventurous soul? Certainly literature is replete with stories of celebrated pilgrims and pathfinders who faced and surmounted harrowing circumstances with legendary resourcefulness and grace.

But you don't need to be a professional hero to act like one when the chips are down. As nearly everyone—adventurer or accountant, mountaineer or office manager—who has faced a crisis and lived to tell *will* tell you, pure calm is often precisely what arises within oneself when circumstances are at their most dire.

Rising to the Occasion

In my life I have known numerous "ordinary" people who have faced acute crises of the most dramatic nature. In some instances, their houses have literally burned to the ground or been shattered by earthquake. Some of these people, indeed probably most of them, would never have supposed themselves the sort to act decisively and constructively in mid-apocalypse. Yet when their respective moments of truth arose, they were able to act with confidence, clarity, and self-command. They rescued themselves, their children, their cats and parakeets, salvaged their prescription glasses, and snagged their kids' favorite stuffed animals as everything else around them crumbled.

Then, too, there are the countless numbers of people who have weathered, with far more courage and resilience than they would ever have foreseen, commonplace life crises (less *dramatic,* but equally *traumatic*) such as divorce, or financial reversals, or the loss of a loved one, or the contraction of a serious illness.

Crises are a part of life. (As one of Tennessee Williams's characters said, "We all live in a house on fire, no fire department to call.") Arguably, though, they are a valuable and necessary part. For as another playwright, Eugène Ionesco, said, "All history is nothing but a succession of 'crises' . . . When there is no 'crisis,' there is stagnation, petrification, and death."

Each of us probably has already faced numerous crises in the course of our existence. Most of us were probably better at facing them—braver, saner, and yes, calmer—than we would ever have dared to hope. But we rarely, if ever, think about how we did it, and from where we drew our strength. And so we miss the significance of crisis, opting instead to anxiously try and prevent another one from occurring in the future.

The Anticrisis

Since the dawn of civilization, humankind—and its collective Busy Mind—has been irresistibly drawn to the enticing idea that circumstances might be controlled and disasters averted if only the right approach could be found. Each culture, in each era, develops crisis-proofing techniques.

In earlier times, sacrifices were made to gods and spirits in the hopes that, as a quid pro quo, droughts or floods might end, battles might be won, and plagues and pestilence be vanquished. Nowadays we tend to invoke insurance agents and lawyers instead of spirits, spending vast sums of money and energy trying to ensure our future security.

We eagerly purchase policies meant to offset our losses in the event of this calamity or that catastrophe. We instigate lawsuits to seek remuneration for every ill that befalls us. And even though the nature of life is, as philosopher Alan Watts said, "the unknown coming into being," we anxiously attempt to think of—and make provisions for—every conceivable worst-case scenario before it happens. (Prenuptial agreements, anyone? One couple gained national notoriety when they filed with their county clerk's office a sixteen-page document specifying not only when they would have children and how often they would make love, but also detailing such marital minutiae as how much they would spend on groceries and what brand of gas they would put in their car.)

But, of course, not every worst case *is* conceivable. You can make an educated guess about what may happen down the road. But can you really know? No.

Despite Henry Kissinger's famed quip—"There can't be a crisis next week. My schedule is already full," crisis sneaks up on you. Without warning, it bursts the fragile balloon of your "safe" world. *That's why they call it a crisis.* You can be as painstakingly cautious and apprehensive as you like, but the gods give no guarantees, and neither do the lawyers.

Deep down, we all know uncertainty to be a fact of life. Yet most of us actively choose to live in denial of this incontrovertible truth. It is a sad irony. Because the idea that we can foresee and prevent all crises is another illusion that enslaves us. It keeps us constantly nervous, hesitant, and on the defensive. What's more, it keeps us so preoccupied with dreaming up interventions to head off troubles that we fail to recognize how the interventions themselves can sometimes lead to even graver woes. (Can you imagine, for example, how many bitter quarrels about prenuptial agreements have dealt wedding plans a terminal blow?)

Life is so complex, its multiple aspects so subtly linked, that we cannot possibly know the effect of one tiny "preventative" action on the larger picture unless, of course, we are omnipotent. And as you may have noticed, despite our occasional grandiose pretensions to the contrary, we do not and cannot—and indeed would not really want to—know everything.

Obviously, no rational person wants to deliberately court trouble and trauma. And you'll be pleased to know that incorporating the Key of Crisis into your life does not involve throwing caution to the winds, emptying out bank accounts, ripping up insurance policies, and firing your attorney, all in the hopes that a crisis will find you and test your mettle.

Crisis finds us all sooner or later. And we must recognize it for the teacher it is. Indeed, we hardly have a choice but to heed its lessons because it demands our full attention. When you're in mid-inferno, you don't stop to call your Allstate agent to buy more fire insurance.

It's just you and the flames. No intermediaries.

Understanding the Key of Crisis

The Third Key to Calm, the Key of Crisis says: *View each crisis as a crash course in calm.* So, just what do we learn in Crisis 101?

Think back over your life to a time when a traumatic incident occurred. Think back to a time when you found strength and resourcefulness you never knew you possessed. Remember when you literally had the thought "I cannot go on," but on you went. I'm going to bet you already learned a few things from that event. For example:

- that it is possible to be free of a sense of your own limits when you are vividly in the moment
- that when you go down the path without a definite plan, doors open along the way
- that your intuition is keener than you expected
- that your priorities can be straightened out in a hurry
- that there seems to be a source of natural power that you can draw on for replenishment when you really need it

You learned these things but, alas, if you're like most of us, you have probably forgotten that you learned them. When the apex of your crisis passed, you began to go back to your old ways of thinking and being. (Proving Richard Nixon was right when he said, "The easiest period in a crisis situation is actually the battle itself.")

Even with the benefit of prior experience, you are probably now doubtful that you could handle another life disruption with similar aplomb. You figure: "That was an exception and not the rule. Next time I'll be a wreck."

But displaying mastery when life throws you a curve ball *can* be the rule, if you let it be.

For the truth is that in order to successfully survive your past crises you automatically accessed the Calm Mind and put the Busy Mind on hold. Once you've done this, the Calm Mind will always be part of your psychic database.

The Polish journalist Ryszard Kapuscinski wrote, "When is a crisis reached? When questions arise that can't be answered." That's as good a definition as any I've ever encountered. We say we are in crisis when we face a situation in which none of the previous patterns we have learned to rely on apply.

Yet somehow we plow through the crisis, improvising as we go, discovering new things about ourselves and about life we never would have otherwise known. We discover that, one way or another, we find the answers to any challenge the universe gives us.

Maybe *that's why it gives them to us!*

The Key of Crisis in Action

Once you begin to consider the possibility that life's crises serve as agents of our mental, emotional, and spiritual education, then the fact that crises are inevitable will not be so anxiety provoking. And once you begin to acknowledge that the Calm Mind "kicks in" in crisis, you will be better able to draw upon its infinite adaptability and wisdom—not just at peak crisis moments, but at all times.

Such beginnings are tenuous. You'll keep being drawn back to old fantasies that you can, with enough anxious forethought, keep crisis at bay. But with the right attitude you will abandon such illusions and the anxieties they bring along with them like so much overstuffed baggage.

What is that right attitude? It can be summed up in one word: surrender.

Of course the word *surrender* may evoke all kinds of negative associations. We may visualize a bedraggled soldier stumbling across a battlefield, feebly brandishing a white flag that signifies "I give up." But consider another meaning of the term.

In the great spiritual traditions of East and West, the concept of surrender is not meant to connote hopelessness or apathy. It is meant to convey *the yielding of the individual will to the ongoing, irrepressible flow of life.* It comes with letting go of fixed ideas about what should be and what will be. It is <u>the acceptance that what is, is.</u>

Keep that definition of surrender in mind. And at a certain point each day (preferably close to waking, or just before retiring), try this simple exercise. Stand or sit in a "receptive" position, that is with your arms outstretched and palms turned up. Then silently think the words "I surrender."

Now your Busy Mind will balk when you first do this. "Oh yeah," it will say none too pleasantly, "you surrender to what?" Let your Calm Mind answer simply: "To Something."

To "Something"?

Yes. Because there is Something (and it doesn't matter what you call it—Fate, God, the Flow of Experience, or, if you prefer *Star Wars* lingo, the Force) more powerful than us. But Something is also somehow part of us and we are somehow part of it.

True, it is this Something that threw you those curve balls that disrupted your life so drastically. But it is also this Something you instinctively tapped into for sustenance. And it is this Something that, without your even thinking about it, helps you combat genuine dangers you aren't even consciously aware you face.

In actuality, each of us confronts many more potential crises in the course of a single day than the most zealous insurance underwriter ever factored into an actuarial table. Sure, sometimes you get sick, but most of the time Something keeps your immune system humming nicely along while you do, let's say, the crossword puzzle or the laundry. Sure, sometimes you have a car crash, but most days Something keeps your car from veering off the road even when your Busy Mind wanders and you're not paying the slightest bit of conscious attention to your driving.

A daily acknowledgment that there is indeed Something to surrender *to* and that you cannot know for sure what this Something has in store will take you all of five seconds to accomplish. But its cumulative impact can yield great composure, because as dusk follows day, calm follows surrender.

Now I realize that performing this exercise in a formal manner just doesn't suit everyone. And if it doesn't fit your style, that's all right. Alternatively, take at least a few moments each day, informally and in a manner of your own choosing, to reflect on the sheer *silliness* of thinking you can make everything in your life turn out just the way you want. You'll find the beneficial effects of this approach to be much the same.

I remember, for example, a gentleman who participated in a psychotherapy group I conducted. He complained that he simply could not get to sleep at night, no matter what he tried. In sessions he often yawned his way through the entire hour. Frustrated, others in the group began to offer him home remedy ideas from hot baths to chamomile tea to calcium-laden bedtime shakes. One night, he finally "confessed" what was keeping him up. He felt as if he had to stay awake, he told the group, in order that he wouldn't lose control over his life. At that point, someone asked him how much control, in the final analysis, he actually had over his life when he was awake. He sat silently for a minute or two and astutely replied, "None." Then he burst out laughing. That night, he later reported, he slept like a stone.

The lesson is clear: in relinquishing the fantasy that you can control all events in life you gain enhanced control over the one thing you truly can master—your own reactions and responses to events.

*I*n our society, most of us would probably define fate as the extent to which the world jerks us around. But it is not fate that unnerves us so much as our own refusal to believe in it. If you truly let crisis be your crash course in calm, you will rapidly learn that it can be fatal to resist fate. (Struggle against a riptide and, poof, you're fish food.) On the other hand, to really accept fate—and the occasional crises it brings—is hardly to be fatalistic. It is to be prepared, always and continually, for change.

For those who wish to overcome anxiety, this is the handiest of traits. For, as you shall see in the next key, the Key of Cycles, understanding and accepting the nature of change is a major part of what separates the calm from the not-so-calm.

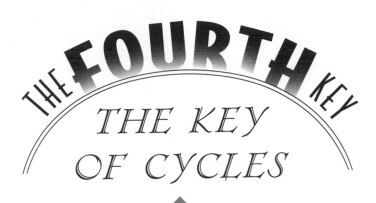

THE FOURTH KEY

THE KEY OF CYCLES

◆

CELEBRATE CHANGE, BECAUSE
CHANGE IS ALL THERE IS.

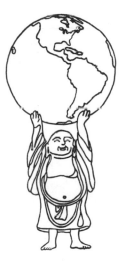

*M*an was made for Joy and Woe
And when this we rightly know
Thro the World we safely go . . .

—WILLIAM BLAKE,
"Auguries of Innocence"

*H*ere or henceforward it is all the same
  to me,
I accept Time absolutely.

—WALT WHITMAN,
"Song of Myself"

THE FOURTH KEY TO CALM

I work with a woman who has diagnosed her greatest anxiety problem as the Full Gas Tank Syndrome. Here's how she describes it:

I never can feel at peace unless I have the sense that everything in the past is resolved and everything in the future looks rosy. I never like to set off on a drive, for example, unless I have just gassed up the car so the tank is brimming. The trouble is, once I start to drive, the gas gauge needle begins to drop. And then I worry, how far can I get on this tank of gas? When should I fill it up again? I can't tell you how much time and energy I waste wishing that everything would just "get done" and remain that way—that the tank would just stay full forever.

Now this is a very bright woman, who sees precisely the paradox she faces. The only way to get the gas tank to stay full eternally, of course, would be to never go anywhere. But standing still is not an option. Like all of us, she has places to go, things to do. And like all of us, she must come to terms with the fact that life—and therefore change—goes on.

Full and Empty, Back and Forth, Up and Down

Cycles of change are everywhere. The tides come in and go out. The moon waxes and wanes. And, as even those of you who may not be nature buffs have probably noticed, interest rates rise and fall, and the stock market grows bearish, then bullish.

Our own bodies are constantly engaging in cycles. Our skin sheds and regenerates; our blood circulates; our bladders fill and demand to be emptied. Without paying much attention, we inhale and exhale numerous times in the course of each minute.

Change is inevitable—a law of the universe. In fact, it is hardly an overstatement to say change is *the* law of the universe. Subatomic quanta—the stuff of which all matter is made—shift from particles to waves and back again. Everything is metamorphosing, all of the time. All is process and flux.

It stands to reason then that to feel at home in the world, one must feel at home with change. To be composed and at ease, one must accept that the only permanent thing is impermanence. Alas, most of us anxiously struggle against change. Instead of feeling at one with it, we stubbornly resist it.

At Odds with Change

We think we are being very clever and tricky in the ways we try to subvert change. Sometimes we try to *deny* change; other times we attempt to *defy* it.

A common tactic for trying to deny change goes something like this: We consider our lot in life, and evaluate its deficiencies. "Life would be pretty good if only this or that would change," we think. ("If only I had more money," for example. Or "If only I could lose ten pounds.") We then proceed to torture ourselves by anxiously obsessing about what we want, wishing for it, fantasizing about getting it, and envying and resenting others who we imagine already have what we want.

The catch is that when we are in this Busy Mindset, we *do* very little to impact positively and influence change. We refuse to work *with* the dynamic of change and take constructive action. Instead, we convince ourselves that, despite evidence to the contrary, *nothing will ever change.* So we opt to mope instead of daring to hope.

Conversely, a common tactic for attempting to defy change works like this: We go along day to day and then suddenly, something especially wonderful befalls us. We get something we've had our heart set on for a long time (that promotion let's say, or a marriage proposal from the love of our life). So what do we do?

We go into a mild panic. "This good fortune can't last," we tell ourselves. "Sooner or later, something is bound to change." We become anxiously preoccupied with imagining exactly what sorts of disasters jealous "gods" or other petty entities might have in store for us, once our proverbial party is over. Then we begin racking our Busy Minds for ways in which we can undermine the natural flow of things and keep circumstances precisely as they are forevermore.

We rehearse over and over again ways of explaining our good fortune to our friends and relations (and even to ourselves) so that it does not seem quite so good after all. We get a wee bit obsessed with knocking on wood and not stepping on cracks. We attempt to make ourselves as inconspicuous as possible so as not to attract attention, as if we could become invisible and make time stand still.

Freud wrote that our possibilities for happiness are "restricted by our constitution." You can clearly see what he means. Having an opportunity for happiness fall into our lap, our first response typically is to dread not having that exact happiness always. We cancel out all the joy of the moment by trying—in vain—to defy change and freeze-frame one moment for all eternity.

It calls to mind the story of a man who believed

that each of us is allotted only a certain number of breaths in life and so decided that by holding his breath he could live forever. Guess how well *that* strategy worked.

The fact is that no matter how hard we work at it, and no matter how much nervous energy we devote, change will not be denied and cannot be defied. We can wallow in hopelessness, saying, "Things will never change." We can anxiously invoke every superstition known to humankind and plead with the cosmos, "Pretty please, don't let anything alter." But that pesky, restless cosmos persists in rearranging things, and neither the "things" themselves nor the emotions and attitudes they evoke in us will ever be anything but impermanent.

Like it or not, change is always with us and within us. So what if, for a change (so to speak), we actively chose to like it?

Understanding the Key of Cycles

The Fourth Key to Calm, the Key of Cycles says: *Celebrate change, because change is all there is.*

By *not* embracing change, we create high levels

of anxiety *because we persist in perceiving as perilous the most fundamental and ubiquitous aspect of the world we inhabit.* Since life *is* change, to be continually anxious in the face of change is to contract a bad case of "lifephobia."

Acrophobics, who fear heights, might be able to construct a life without venturing onto too many bridges and mountaintops. Hydrophobics, who fear water, might be able to exist quite tolerably while remaining recalcitrantly landlocked. But can a "lifephobic" avoid life?

Lots of us try.

By persisting in equating feelings of calm and security exclusively with fixity and permanence, we are distancing ourselves from life. It's as if we are trying our damnedest to stay rooted to one spot while situated on a racing locomotive. We are missing the entire point, not to mention the entire ride.

Ironically, the sense of incongruity that results from trying vainly to embrace two distinctly opposed concepts actually *increases* our feelings of insecurity. The more we believe only permanence will "save" us, the more jittery we are bound to become as such permanence continually eludes us.

If we were to genuinely pay attention and bring

awareness to the situation, we would have to admit to ourselves the obvious. True peace and calm can be attained only by acquiescing to change and by staying flexible in the face of life's fluidity.

You probably haven't given it much thought, but consider for a minute what existence would be like if nothing around you progressed and changed. Let's say you could press a "pause" button on your life right now and keep your finger holding it down. There would be no more music or dancing, of course, because there would be only one note playing monotonously on and on. You'd never get to see the sun set, since it wouldn't. You could forget about running water, since it couldn't. Besides all that, no one would ever pick up your trash again. And your toddlers would never graduate from their Huggies Pull-Ups phase.

Oh, boy.

Now obviously this is anything but a calming scenario. It's more like an episode of *The Twilight Zone.* But it is the logical extension of what so many of us *think* we want. Its eeriness and ridiculousness are worth pondering when we feel ourselves denying or resisting inevitable change.

The Key of Cycles in Action

Embracing change, and celebrating it, is no effortless task. Because of the way our Busy Mind thinks, perhaps nothing is as easy to advise and as hard to do as "going with the flow." But here's the good news: In the course of evolution, only those who adapted as circumstances altered survived and thrived. It's fair to say that not one of us would be here now if we weren't fundamentally capable of change at the deepest of levels. And at such a primordial level, the Calm Mind holds sway.

To translate the Key of Cycles into action, we need, once again, to allow our Calm Mind to play a role. The Calm Mind does not concern itself with fearing future changes or regretting past ones, because it is always *in the moment*. And because it is always in the moment, it is totally able to respond to exactly what is happening as it happens.

The Calm Mind accepts life's ups and downs, not because it is philosophically resigned, but because it is instinctively moving along with them. One might say the Calm Mind doesn't experience ups and downs as such, but instead experiences each instant of every incline or decline as just that one instant. Riding the wave from crest to trough, it is at one with the wave.

There is an old Zen parable about a man who is being chased by a tiger. To evade the beast, the man jumps off the edge of a cliff and clings to a vine. Climbing down the vine, he spies another tiger below. The vine begins to break. The man notices a strawberry growing on the side of the cliff, which he plucks and enjoys.

Now imagine the Busy Mind in such a situation. Its deafening chatter would probably go something like: "Yikes, that was close. Omigosh, what's gonna happen now? Oh gee, it's another tiger. I bet he'll chase me too. I'm sure he will. I wish he wouldn't. I wish I'd stayed in bed. Woe is me. Oh, please, God or Someone in Charge—I just want to hang here forever. Now the vine is tearing? Give me a break! I'm doomed!" Whether or not the second tiger gives chase, of course, this Busy Mind is indeed doomed. It is doomed always to miss out on the good things life has to offer.

In a way, each of us is suspended between perils. As the late Gilda Radner liked to remind us, sooner or later, "It's always something." But what if we, like our trusty Zen traveler, were able to *no-*

tice and experience just one valuable thing in any given situation rather than fearing what might or might not happen next?

The next time you catch yourself obsessively wishing that circumstances would change only in a particular way or praying they will never again change at all, gently usher yourself out of the trap you have set for yourself. Do this by looking for and focusing on something worthwhile that is right in front of you—the "strawberry."

Suppose there is no strawberry, you say? Suppose I am in a situation where there is nothing whatsoever worthwhile.

But what situation could have no strawberry at all? Of course, you may not literally chance across a tasty delicacy to delight in every time you're feeling anxious about the future. But many things other than sensual pleasures are worthy of commanding our full attention.

Try looking at each situation with curiosity. Is there anything in your immediate circumstance about which you could learn and understand more? Begin to observe and study that thing, and your Busy Mind will quiet down.

Try looking at your situation with creativity. Is

there something that could inspire you to write, to draw, to make music? As Paul Cézanne advised, "Right now, a moment in time is fleeting by! Capture its reality in paint! To do that we must put all else out of our minds."

Try looking around you with compassion. In your immediate circumstance, do you notice anyone who could use your understanding or encouragement? Then make yourself useful. Remember the Second Key to Calm: Assisting someone—anyone—in precisely the way they need to be assisted is an excellent way of grounding oneself in the now and keeping the Busy Mind from dwelling on what may or may not happen next.

Even in the bleakest of situations, try looking at what surrounds you with an open, nonjudgmental Calm Mind and you will probably see that there is always something worthwhile to focus on with awareness, something to appreciate. Even our pains and troubles can be appreciated for instructing and strengthening us. And even they are less frightening when we are willing to observe them rather than struggle against them.

Make no mistake, immersing yourself in the moment will not prevent change. And fear not, your newfound ability will not rob you of your powers to make certain prudent plans for the future, based on educated guesses. Your awareness of "strawberries," however, will help you to be detached from your anxiety concerning life's continual vacillations and transitions. What's more, it will help you make the most of the many opportunities that transitions offer. For where there is infinite change, there is infinite possibility.

*T*he Key of Cycles is about letting yourself dance the dance and sing the song, without fast-forwarding your brain to the final note. It must also be said that part of being human is being conscious of the fact that someday, at some point, all of our songs and all of our dances—as we now know them—will encounter an ultimate transition from life to whatever lies beyond life. For the undeniable, inherently logical extension of the law of change is that change and mortality are inseparable bedfellows.

Now you may hardly consider this a calming thought, and not wish to be reminded of it. However, in the Fifth Key to Calm, the Key of Cessation, you will see how the inevitability of death—the ultimate change—can help, rather than hinder us, in our continuing search for serenity.

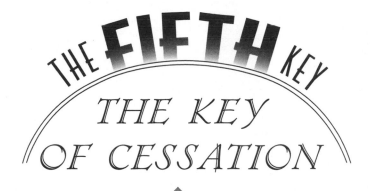

THE FIFTH KEY

THE KEY OF CESSATION

◆

MAKE AN ALLY OF YOUR
MORTALITY.

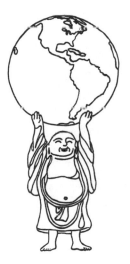

*B*e cheerful, sir.
Our revels now are ended. These our
  actors,
As I foretold you, were all spirits, and
Are melted into air, into thin air.
                              —WILLIAM SHAKESPEARE,
                                          The Tempest

*L*et us deprive death of its strangeness;
let us frequent it, let us get used to it; let
us have nothing more often in mind than
death . . . To practice death is to practice
freedom.

                              —MICHEL DE MONTAIGNE,
                                          Essays

THE FIFTH KEY TO CALM

One day a young woman stormed into my office, twenty minutes late for a session and as anxious and frustrated as could be. Grumbling and grousing, Meredith recounted a long string of acute annoyances that had served to make her day a highly stressful and unpleasant one. She'd been locked out of her apartment by her roommate, her subway train had gotten stuck between stops, one of those little screws on the temple piece of her eyeglass frame had fallen out, and—indignity of indignities—an automated teller machine had devoured her bank card.

She went on and on about her complaints, working herself up into quite a lather. "Life sucks, and then you die," she explained. Then she added, "Oh well, at least after I die, I won't have to deal with automated teller machines."

"How do you know?" I asked her.

She thought about that a second, and then it seemed my comment, which had been meant to prod Meredith out of her redundant complaining, succeeded. Her foul mood dispelled by laughter, Meredith spent the rest of her therapy session on a more philosophical bent.

What did she know about death, she mused? Like the rest of us, nothing much. Only that it probably wasn't going to be business as usual. Only that it would likely render the attachments and aversions we so carefully cultivate in this world (e.g., our cravings for sex, money, and Ben & Jerry's; our grudges against automated teller machines and public transportation) wholly beside the point. Only that the mystery of death had the power to make one look at one's day-to-day existence from an entirely new perspective.

"I'm amazed," said Meredith, "that I never really thought about death this way before."

But in this, of course, she is far from alone.

"Deathphobia"

In our society, very few of us devote much mental energy to pondering death, or its implications for life. Intellectually, we know we will someday make the journey to what Shakespeare called "the undiscovered country." But emotionally, either we use this fact as another reason to suffer anxiety, or we march headlong into denial. What we "know" we do not really accept.

Many other cultures throughout history have integrated death into their view of life in a psychologically and spiritually beneficial manner. Through religious and mystical beliefs, along with the attitudes and rituals such beliefs brought into existence, their psychic infrastructure incorporated death's reality rather than trying to suppress and evade it. Death was respected as the completion of a cycle, a return to the state in which we existed before we were born.

In other times and in other places, death was

bound up with the sacred. But in turn-of-the-millennium America, we seem to have gotten things scrambled. Talk of death, or anything having to do with death, gives us the heebie-jeebies. It's as if we, as a society, have made a psychic "typo" on a grand scale: we've rearranged the letters in *sacred*—and gotten just plain *scared*.

Walk through a bookstore or health food store, or wander past a cosmetics counter today, and what do you see? An ever-widening range of tomes and pills and creams that promise us the secrets of "anti-aging." Good deal, we think. No aging, well . . . maybe no *you-know-what*.

But, hey, even if we can't forestall *you-know-what* indefinitely, maybe we can look into those proliferating cryogenics services which, for a fee, will store our bodies (or just our heads if we prefer) in liquid nitrogen. Then, in the event that future scientific methods may someday enable us to book a passage back from the Beyond, we will return little worse for the wear (though perhaps in need of a facial and a sun lamp).

Certainly we all share an understandable reluctance to let go of the powerful ties that bind us to this existence. Indeed, none other than Timothy

Leary—once world famous for his adventurous journeying into other realms—was quoted as asking, when he first learned he had a terminal illness and was planning his own cryogenic stasis, "Why let the carefully arranged tangle of dendritic growths in your nervous system which store all your memories get eaten by fungus?"

But, as this traveler came to see, and as all we travelers must come to understand, the real question concerning death is not *why* but, as Leary's very last words, reported by a friend at his bedside were, "Why not?"

Because death is part of life. Because all things that take form ultimately dissolve and all things that begin ultimately end. And, most of all, because—*until we are reconciled with these truths, we will never be really at peace.*

Understanding the Key of Cessation

The Fifth Key to Calm, the Key of Cessation (*cessation* literally meaning "going from action to rest") says: *Make an ally of your mortality.*

When we really think about death—without considering it an enemy to be vanquished, that is—a lot of amazing things can happen. It can alter profoundly what we choose to spend our time on, what we think is important, what we truly value, and what's worth worrying about and what's not. Indeed, for all that gives life meaning, we have our mortal cessation to thank.

Do you recall the classic play *Our Town,* by Thornton Wilder? (You probably read it back in high school English class.) In it, a young woman, Emily, who dies after giving birth to her second child, asks to go back and relive just one day of her life in the simple town of Grover's Corners.

Emily's wish is granted, but what she finds is not what she expected. The humdrum details of everyday life—the smell of coffee, the ticking of clocks, the look of sunflowers, the feel of a hot bath or a freshly ironed dress—overwhelm her with their richness and beauty. So do the relationships between her and the people she loved. "Oh, earth," laments Emily, "you're too wonderful for anybody to realize you."

Through her tears she asks the Stage Manager (the character who appears to administer the realms of life and death), "Do any human beings ever realize life while they live it?—every, every minute?"

"No," the Stage Manager replies.

And, of course, he is right. None of us can be aware and awake *every* minute. As another character among *Our Town*'s dead says, most of us in the realm of the living tend to "move about in a cloud" and are "always at the mercy of some self-centered passion, or another." There are, however, a few among us who manage to "realize life," as Wilder so eloquently puts it, much of the time.

For example, in his book, *Thoughts Without a Thinker,* Mark Epstein, a psychotherapist and practicing Buddhist, tells of visiting a monk named Achaan Chaa at a Thailand monastery. One day, the monk gave a lesson. He picked up a plain drinking goblet and explained that, to him, it was beautiful. It held water adequately, reflected the light when held up to the sun, and rang out prettily when tapped. But, really, the goblet was most beautiful to him because it was "already broken." The fact that at some point the glass was destined to fall from a shelf or be brushed off the table by an errant elbow and shatter into fragments is precisely what made it so worth cherishing.

What if each of us were to try, each day, if not every minute than at least for a few moments, to employ this point of view? What if we were to reflect on the reality that everything—the glasses we drink from, the chairs we sit on, the books we read to ourselves, and indeed *even our very selves*—are destined "to break"?

Well, that's morbid, you say. But is it? Think about watching a young infant at play, smiling and cooing, rhapsodizing over a rattle. We watch this and our hearts feel full to overflowing. Not just because the baby is adorable and lovable. But because, deep down, we understand that this baby's babyhood is fleeting by and soon will no longer exist. Where the tiny baby was, something else will be. A toddler, a schoolchild, an adolescent, an adult.

That is the way things are. And though we are all here now, someday, someone else will be in our place. Like many societies who went before ours, or who coexist with ours in other places on this planet, we could actively *choose* to label this reality not as morbid but as sacred.

If we did so choose, then our seemingly ceaseless anxieties about *getting more of this* or *getting rid of that* would be put to rest—because all ordinary things would seem extraordinary and we would value what we had. Then we would stop trying to "fix" everybody and everything—because we would understand that there isn't anything we can permanently fix. Then we would stop obsessing on predicting and controlling outcomes—because we would already know and accept the ultimate outcome.

With many of our anxieties thus quelled, we would free up enormous sums of energy to make the best use of this life while we still have the opportunity to do so.

The Key of Cessation in Action

But what is the best use of life and of our own life energy? I'm reminded of the boy who comes home from school having acquired the knowledge that the sun is going to go supernova in a billion or so years and asks, "So why do I have to do my homework?" We, too, often seem to wonder: What's the point?

In our recent history, the predominant answer has seemed to be: The point is to acquire a lot of things. Or, as one popular 1980s bumper sticker put it: WHOEVER DIES WITH THE MOST TOYS WINS.

But acquisition is really a goal of the Busy Mind, which wants to insulate itself by accumulating things which, it believes, will act as barriers between itself and unwanted emotions such as fear and worry. Yet having exclusively material goals in life only *increases* our anxiety level.

Two Zen parables illustrate how too much attachment to material goods can undermine peace of mind:

In the first, a farmer finds a priceless gold statue, reputedly one of nineteen gold icons. His friends and family are overjoyed. But immediately the farmer starts worrying: Where are the other eighteen?

In the second, a famous general is polishing an antique cup that is very dear to him. He nearly drops it and becomes frantic. He wonders why he can fearlessly lead soldiers into battle, yet be terrorized by this tiny teacup. When he realizes how much his attachment rules him, he throws the teacup over his shoulder and shatters it.

When I came across these stories, I couldn't help recalling the old George Carlin routine, in which the comedian makes fun of our propensity for gathering "stuff." We buy a house and fill it with stuff. Then we get so much stuff we fret that we need a bigger house. If we go on vacation, we obsess on how much stuff we can bring with us. And if while on vacation we embark on a day trip, we cram as much of our traveling stuff as possible into tote bags, knapsacks and king-size handbags.

Now I like stuff as much as the next red-blooded American consumer, and there's nothing wrong with enjoying nice things. I obtain, for example, enormous pleasure and satisfaction from typing these very words on my trusty, efficient, easy-to-operate Macintosh PowerPC. But, let's face it, when my time comes to move on, wherever it is that I'm going, my Macintosh is not coming with me. So, while I appreciate it, I try not to overvalue it, or fret that I need a better, faster, newer model *now*. Like all of us, I have to take care to remind myself that ultimate satisfaction in life cannot be derived from a computer, or a car, or anything I claim to possess.

It's ironic that many people even use acquisition as a means of countering their fear of death itself. Getting and spending may offer the illusion of immortality for a brief moment, but such a strategy is doomed to backfire because much of our fear of death can be fear of parting with things to which we are attached, and things that we perceive as "belonging" to us. *Yet nothing actually belongs to us.*

On the ultimate journey one packs light and customs regulations are strict. You can't take anything with you. Not your designer luggage, not your American Express card, not your physical body, not your opinions, attitudes, feelings or busy thoughts.

Though it may not appear so at first, this truth actually points us in the direction of calm. For once we accept that we actually own nothing, we realize we have nothing to lose. What's more, we now have everything to give.

Now the real point of what we are doing here—if we are all going to die anyway—becomes clear. If we can't take anything with us, the point must lie in what we can leave behind. So what, exactly, can we leave?

All physical things erode—even the house and jewelry we may will to our descendants; even the vital organs we may donate to a sufferer of illness.

Ultimately, then, the point lies less in what we give than in what spirit we give it.

As the Buddha said, neither fire nor wind, birth nor death, can erase our good deeds. The one thing, the only thing that can be our everlasting legacy is our *positive intent,* that is, the selfless acts we have performed on behalf of others out of unconditional acceptance and love.

To put the Key of Cessation into action, we need to begin to prioritize what we do and how we expend our energy in the context of positive intent. In modern life we are anxiously torn between so many tasks. We are pressured to accrue more and more, and achieve more and more. In addition, we are made to feel that unless we do everything expertly (work out until we have the ideal body; emulate Martha Stewart so we can make a breathtaking centerpiece from sock lint and twine), we are somehow insufficient. Unsure which of these activities, if any, will bring us the sense of peace and fulfillment we crave, we stretch ourselves to the breaking point attempting to "pack it all in" so that we can be sure we are "really living."

But if you let your mortality advise you, your sense of frantic urgency will diminish. Think about it. When you have left this life, this body, what bit of your essence do you want to survive you? What memories do you wish to leave people with? Picture a memorial service where friends, colleagues, and relations stand up and say, "This was a guy who always checked his E-mail," or "He drove a cool car and waxed it compulsively." How about: "She was always able to find a bargain." Some legacy.

But how about: "He was never too tired to read bedtime stories to his kids," or "She was never too busy to listen," or "This was one fellow who knew how to appreciate the little things in life—and who knew how to make us all laugh." That sounds more like it.

For when it's all said and done, such efforts resonate eternally, with one positive intention inspiring another and another, ad infinitum. (This is *karma*—or universal cause and effect—in the truest sense.)

Obviously, not all of life can be spent executing good works. And not every moment will be spent actively appreciating life's bounty. Bills must be paid, phones answered, lists compiled and dutifully checked off. Such is the upkeep of our day-to-day lives. But keeping the goal of positive intent in mind helps us focus, helps us make choices, and helps us separate the wheat from the chaff. It helps us remain calm, too. Because we realize "having it all" and "doing it all" are not worth worrying about. And because fear of death turns to respect for death when one concentrates on living with positive intent.

So the next time you are frazzled by the prospect of too many chores, too many commitments, too many goals, try using the following method to settle on which activity to focus on. Ask yourself: *If this next hour were my last on earth, how would I choose to spend it?* Or: *Which of these things would I most like to be remembered for?* Then pursue your choice wholeheartedly.

A Note on Afterlife

Having said this much about death, it would be a grievous omission not to note that many people believe in a rebirth of sorts after death. Some strongly believe in the eventuality of rebirth in Heaven, and are greatly reassured by this conviction.

Others believe they will reincarnate again on

earth. This belief, too, for the millions and millions who subscribe to it, can offer profound emotional sustenance. As Henry Ford, who came to believe avidly in this prospect, put it, "When I discovered reincarnation . . . I was no longer a slave to the hands of the clock. . . . I would like to communicate to others the calmness that the long view of life gives to us."

Much silliness and nonsense has been perpetrated around the concept of reincarnation. (It is, for example, unlikely that as many of us as claim to actually preexisted as Indian princesses or members of Egyptian royalty.) It could be argued as well that some popular notions of an afterlife life in Heaven (wherein we are all handed harps and halos at the door and spend eternity floating about on cloud wisps) also seem somewhat romanticized. It's understandable, therefore, that some people remain skeptical about an afterlife. Besides, doubters say, belief in an afterlife is not based on scientific fact, and so is not "logical."

But in the great scheme of things, who's to say what's really logical? As Voltaire philosophized, "It's no more surprising to be born twice than to be born once." As Candace Pert, a world-renowned brain researcher, posited, "Matter can neither be created nor destroyed, and perhaps biological information flow cannot just disappear at death and must be transformed into another realm." Besides, as Woody Allen noted, the idea that there may be no afterlife can be "a depressing thought, particularly for those who have bothered to shave."

Still and all, no one can *make* you believe in an afterlife. And such belief is not necessary in order to put the Fifth Key to Calm into effect. Whether you believe you will live in Heaven, live again on earth, or be reborn simply as a part of the grass that grows, prioritizing your earthly existence in terms of positive intent will soothe and quiet you as you progress through this life and as you approach its natural end.

Unlike all other earthly things, positive intent is not "here today, gone tomorrow." With positive intent as your legacy, you will have penned your signature across the scrolls of eternity. That is a calming thought if ever there was one.

*T*he theologian Ivan Illich said, "At the moment of death I hope to be surprised." I'd wager his hope will be realized.

Death is a mysterious, creative force. While we are living, we will never have all our questions about it resolved. So be it. We can still "make sense" of death as a teacher, and calm ourselves by doing so. After all, we will never have all of our questions about life resolved either. But, as we will see in the Sixth Key to Calm, we can also "make sense" of life in a way that will serve to alleviate anxiety.

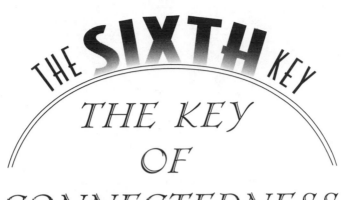

THE **SIXTH** KEY

THE KEY
OF
CONNECTEDNESS

◆

NOTICE THAT LIFE WORKS.

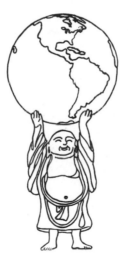

We dance round in a ring and suppose,
But the Secret sits in the middle and
knows.

> —ROBERT FROST,
> "The Secret Sits"

Everything is a miracle. It is a miracle
one does not dissolve in one's bath like a
lump of sugar.

> —PABLO PICASSO

We try to explain the strange in terms
of the familiar, but sometimes it just won't
stop being strange.

> —GEORGE JOHNSON

THE SIXTH KEY TO CALM

*T*here's a day in my life I'll never forget: I was just twenty-one, a freshly minted college graduate. I was in New York City, looking for a job in book publishing, along with a zillion or so similar hopefuls.

I didn't know a soul in the book business, had no friends or contacts to rely on. My only "professional" experience with literature had been a brief stint working at a bookstore. In short, I was as green as a Granny Smith apple.

I answered ads from *The New York Times,* and arrived at interviews clutching a binder full of writing samples. These included regular columns I had written for my college paper and short stories published in college lit magazines. But nobody wanted to see my writing samples. It turned out the interviewers for the positions I was applying for (euphemistically called *entry level*) were actually interested in typing rather than writing ability. And at typing I had only limited success.

Finally, I applied at an employment agency purporting to specialize in the book business. At their behest I set off to a well-known publishing firm to interview as an assistant in what was known as the Traffic Department. The available job, I was told, was for someone who would "work closely with the warehouse" making sure new printings were shipped to stores in a timely fashion. Hardly the glamour I'd anticipated, but I dutifully went forth, still carrying the now increasingly superfluous writing samples.

I was told to go to the twenty-first floor of such-and-such an address and ask for a woman named Judy Wasserman, in Personnel. I exited the elevator at what I thought was the twenty-first floor.

"Judy, uh, Wass . . ." I mumbled to the receptionist, trying to retrieve from my purse the slip of paper with the relevant details. "Uh, I'm here for the job interview."

"Oh," said the receptionist brightly, "you mean Jane Wesman. Down the hall, third door on your left."

Believing, truly, that I was in the right place, I interviewed with this Ms. Wesman for the better part of an hour. She asked me questions about what kind of reading I liked to do, whether I'd enjoy meeting and working closely with authors, and—hallelujah—whether I had any writing samples.

As you probably have already figured out (though I genuinely still had not), I was interviewing for the "wrong" job with the "wrong" person. Judy Wasserman, sitting one floor upstairs in the Personnel Department, was still wondering what had happened to the young woman who was supposed to interview for the trafficking job. But before I left the building, I had a position in the Publicity Department as a book publicist. It was a field I would work happily in for the better part of the next decade.

A happy coincidence? Blind chance? Dumb luck? Call it what you will. But do you want to know something? Virtually everyone I've ever asked has a tale akin to this one to tell.

As much as we are made anxious by the thought of getting things wrong or making mistakes in our lives, virtually all of us are familiar with the experience of stumbling and blundering our way into great good fortune.

Blunders and Blessings

I know a woman who missed a flight that was to have taken her to an important meeting—and then met her husband-to-be as she sat at the airport stewing over her delay. I know a man who was let go from a job—only to dream up the idea for a highly successful business venture with a similarly "downsized" colleague he met on an unemployment line. In my therapy practice I have heard countless stories wherein people, often feeling at their lowest, seem somehow to bump into exactly the right circumstances to resolve their particular problem (though it may take them a while to recognize these "blessings in disguise" as such).

My guess is that each of you reading this book has also experienced a number of astounding coincidences or quirks of fate. They come when you least expect them. They work in circuitous ways. If asked, you'd probably say these are flukes that defy explanation. But throughout the course of history, psychologists, scientists, and mystics have come up with some fascinating theories on their genesis.

Carl Jung, the pioneering Swiss psychoanalyst, spoke of something he termed *synchronicity,* a connecting principle that underlies existence and gives it meaning. (When you are thinking of someone you haven't seen in a long while and your phone rings and it's that person, that's a garden variety of synchronicity.) Jung took synchronicity as evidence that "in all chaos there is a cosmos, in all disorder a secret order."

Many scientists, too, have posited that things that appear disordered might actually conceal order of an infinitely high degree. Quantum physicist David Bohm elaborated on this idea by referring to a device he himself "stumbled" across while watching a BBC television program. The device was a glycerin-filled jar containing a large rotating cylinder at its center. Floating in the thick, clear, liquid glycerin was one drop of ink. Bohm was fascinated to see that when the cylinder was turned by rotating a crank atop the jar, the drop of ink spread throughout the glycerin. As soon as the crank was turned in the opposite direction, however, the ink slowly collapsed on itself, again becoming one droplet. This led Bohm to posit that the ink had a "hidden" order when it was spread out, which was "revealed" when it was reconstituted.

The jar crystallized Bohm's thinking and helped him constitute a theory that had been floating about in his own mind, like so much spread-out ink, for a number of years. The physical universe we perceive, he said, is actually a kind of illusion. Underlying what we see and hear and touch through our ordinary senses is a deep, enfolded order, a more intrinsic level of reality.

Bohm used the metaphor of a hologram to further explain his vision of the universe. Like a piece of holographic film, he said, the universe we experience is actually a sort of projected image. But within each bit of the universe, as within each bit of holographic film, lies the hidden or enfolded whole, the big picture.

How would this explain the astounding coincidences Jung termed synchronicity? Another physicist, David Peat, in his book, *Synchronicity: The Bridge Between Mind and Matter,* theorized that startling, psychologically meaningful coincidences could be explained by Bohm's holographic model. He called such coincidences "flaws in the fabric of reality." They are nothing less than moments, he said, when we get to step outside linear time— suspending our past, present, and future mode of thinking and perceiving—to peek around the corner and see everything revealed at once.

Synchronicities, Peat said, also illustrate that our thought processes themselves are more intimately connected with the physical world than most of us ever imagined. Because consciousness and matter are merely different manifestations of the same unified entity (just dispersed bits of the same droplet of ink, as it were), we actually possess the latent ability to participate in the creation of reality.

Simply put, we may not have simply tripped across business opportunities or found our future fiancés willy-nilly. We may in some way, at certain emotionally charged moments, cause opportunities to be there and cause ourselves to intersect with those opportunities.

Of course, if you are familiar with certain aspects of religion and philosophy, such ideas may not be entirely new to you. For millennia, mystics from traditions as diverse as Hinduism, Buddhism, and Kabbalism (the esoteric interpretation of the Hebrew scriptures) have told us that what we think of as "reality" is nothing more than an illusion, an illusion filtered through our own senses—which fragment the underlying unity of all things. Behind that illusion, they say, is a far more fundamental order of existence, an infinite interconnectedness.

Like today's quantum physicists, who use the hologram as a metaphor to describe the inextricable nature of "here," "there" and "everywhere," mystic sages have compared our universe to a countless array of jewels, each with countless facets reflecting in themselves every other jewel in existence. And like David Peat, those sages have long believed that under certain circumstances we can not only view all the connections and reflections but also influence the array itself.

Now most of us are neither mystics nor quantum physicists, and this sort of theorizing can sometimes be as overwhelming as it is fascinating. Yet, on a gut level, most of us seem to harbor a powerful suspicion that *there is more going on in life than meets the eye,* even if we don't dare say so aloud. And most of us have found ourselves, on occasion, awestruck and humbled by the way one thing or another miraculously seemed to work out just when we most needed it to.

That suspicion, that snippet of awe, is all that's necessary to begin to employ the sixth Key to Calm.

Understanding the Key of Connectedness

The Sixth Key to Calm, the Key of Connectedness, simply states: *Notice that life works.*

It doesn't say notice *why* life works, or even *how* life works. There are certain aspects of the how and why of life that may simply be unknowable. But work it does. And noticing its workings can imbue us with a deep sense of calm. Because what we can't help but notice, if we really pay attention, is that the universe appears to be intelligent, even compassionate.

Notice how many of life's mistakes turn out to be marvels. Think back over the course of your personal path through life and recall those times when you "failed" to fulfill a certain dream, only to have something even better happen—something perhaps that you never even dared to dream of. Think of the times your entire life seemed to be in chaos, but the alleged "chaos," you later discovered, actually contained the seeds of your rightful future. Now think not only of your own history, but of history in a larger context.

Think about the "accidents" that led to some of the world's greatest discoveries. (Like that bit of *Penicillium notatum* fungus that fell into a preparation of bacteria a researcher had been planning to throw away, until he noticed that no bacteria grew where the penicillin had fallen.)

Consider also that the biggest "mistake-maker" on the planet is nothing less than the genetic material from which all life forms are made: the helical molecule of DNA. As the physician Lewis Thomas wrote, "The capacity to blunder slightly is the real marvel of DNA. . . . Viewed individually, one by one, each of the mutations that have brought us along represents a random, totally spontaneous accident, but it is no accident at all that mutations occur; *the molecule DNA was ordained from the beginning to make small mistakes.*" A good thing, as he points out, or you and I would be a couple of anaerobic bacteria.

A good thing too that you and I, who are here by virtue of the existence of DNA—and whatever force or forces may have created and guided *it,* appear to be similarly ordained to pursue a course of trial and error (or, more appropriately put, trial and breakthrough). For if we were confined to a life of certainties, that would be no life at all. We would never experiment, nor would we leave ourselves open for the mysterious forces of synchronicity to work with. And so we would never discover what was really possible.

Notice how life uses messes to make progress. No one can deny that life is messy. And messes tend to make us nervous. Caught in mid-mess, we tend to have the feeling that things can only get worse, that the situation can only deteriorate. But look around, and you will see that such is not the rule.

Hypothetically, a tendency toward inertia and

stagnation takes place in all systems. Disorder and randomness inevitably increase throughout the entire universe, and all matter and energy regress toward a state of inert uniformity. This is what's known as entropy.

Inexplicably, however, life continually counteracts entropy. Atoms bond into molecules of greater and greater complexity. Bacteria do not get to laze around the planet by themselves but have to share it with chameleons, crickets, gazelles, giraffes, morning glories, mako sharks, and, of course, us (who, in turn, play host to diverse populations of countless microbes within our own bodies). Self-sustaining systems abound, and countless species blossom, buzz, and blow about in unison, to their mutual benefit. You need only take a walk in a garden to prove it all to yourself.

At first glance, life may appear drunk and disorderly, downright slatternly. But on closer inspection one notices a method in its madcap shenanigans. Life is full of messes, to be sure, but life actually makes use of them to move forward: forward toward order, forward toward organization, forward toward synchronization.

Like life, we can (and somehow do, even if we

do not mean to) make use of our messes. We can play with them, fiddle with them, and ultimately alchemize them into a prolific, productive outcome.

Notice how life's little pieces fit together. In the course of daily life we tend to view things as sequential and one-dimensional. We see cause and effect as a straight, unbroken chain. For example, we break eggs, add butter, put them in a pan, and make breakfast. End of story. But, if you really think about it, the story of this simple breakfast goes off in all directions at once.

The egg came from a chicken; the chicken ate chickenfeed, and also swallowed stones to grind up its food in its gizzard. The butter was churned from milk, which came from a cow, which ate the grass, which grew with the aid of rainwater. The frying pan came from a store, and before that from a factory. The store and factory were both staffed with people who, without realizing it, were instrumental in helping you cook this modest repast so you could begin your day with some energy. And that energy will carry you through the morning, the morning in which you will do something productive at your job or in your home.

So your deeds of the morning, like your morning meal itself, are in some way cocreated by the combined efforts of nature (in the form of chickens, cows, stones, and rainwater) and human intent (the intent of the factory workers to make a frying pan, the intent of the store workers to sell the frying pan, and your own intent to manifest a scrambled egg on a plate).

Naturally we can't stand at our range tops musing of such things each moment, or we would never get any breakfast at all. But it's great fun—and very useful—to indulge such trains of thought from time to time. For when you do so, you can't help but notice that nothing exists in isolation. Everything is connected to everything else, and everyone to everyone else. Although it would be impossible to ever really understand the complete and unabridged story of what is going on, it's clear something bigger than each of us—and bigger than each of our individual worries and problems and struggles—is *always* going on.

This realization of interconnectedness is shared, in varying degrees, by the world's great prophets, artists, scientists, and statesmen (not to mention many highly successful businessmen). The more one sees it, the more creative one is likely to be, and the calmer one is likely to be, as well.

For though we may grow anxious at times that we are insignificant or that we "don't know what we are doing," we may rest assured that we are doing something. We are sounding our individual note in a vast symphony. And there will be in life fleeting moments—synchronous moments, if you will—when, if we stop and listen, we can hear the perfect harmonies.

The Key of Connectedness in Action

Now you are doing a lot of noticing. But your Busy Mind keeps coming back to *how*s and *why*s.

Why all these "mistakes" and messes? it asks. What are all these intricate connections for, and what—or who—is responsible for them?

In reply, I will tell you a teaching ascribed to the Buddha—who, it is said, cautioned against asking too many questions about the nature of existence. He likened a person who does so to a man who, having been shot by an arrow, refuses to have its sharp point extracted until he knows for sure who shot the arrow, where he was from, what he looked like, and precisely what sort of bow he was using. Needless to say, that man would die before his questions could be answered. The queries would prove pointless, not to mention impractical in the extreme.

Why ask why, after all? No answer could truly satisfy the Busy Mind. For one thing, it would only lead to more questions. "Have I got the whole story now?" the Busy Mind would wonder nervously. "Is there still something I'm missing?" For another thing, it might engender a rigid set of opinions that would then have to be desperately, anxiously clung to and defended. "Your beliefs don't agree with my beliefs," the Busy Mind would say. "Why, you must be dangerous!"

On the other hand, keeping an open mind and remaining open to all possibilities is the ultimate self-calming attitude. For it implies a trust and faith that benevolent forces help maintain us as we wend our way through this world, and that nothing we do—or neglect to do—can obliterate or curtail such forces.

By merely *staying observant to life's workings,* we

see evidence, incontrovertible evidence, of those benevolent forces all around us. And, for reasons I don't purport to understand and don't care to, the more we take note of the universe's benevolent, maintaining forces, the greater the role they seem to play for us. (Perhaps they simply like being appreciated!)

Try it. Spend some time thinking about how one seemingly minor, inconsequential event in your life led to another and another until you ended up in a place that felt like *exactly where you were supposed to be.* Then see what happens. The more you acknowledge the connections, the more frequently synchronicities will manifest themselves in your life—and the more you can relax in the knowledge that your life, at this very moment, is a work in progress, whose outcome will probably be better than you envision.

Troubleshooting

Once again, a word of warning is in order. Even trust in a wise universe can be misused if not tempered with your own individual wisdom.

Do not anticipate that by developing openness

and faith in life's mysterious forces that the endings of your various stories will be like fairy tales, wherein you live happily ever after. No ending is an ending, but only a segue to another beginning. Besides, "happiness" is relative.

The Busy Mind, so anxious to feel satisfied (and so fundamentally incapable of it), imagines happiness is getting all one's needs met all of the time. But a life without hardship, without challenge, and without its share of sorrows would be less a life than a kind of suspended animation. Looking back through life's intricate web of connections, one can't help but concede it is precisely through enduring hardship of one kind or another that one becomes a broader, more evolved being, more capable of understanding and assisting others and of using that sense of compassion to find peace. Try, now and again, to recognize the groundwork for your growth in the hardship *while* you are enduring it, and serenity will be yours.

Also, do not for one moment imagine that trusting in the universe absolves you of personal responsibility. The I-don't-have-to-do-anything-cuz-the-universe-will-take-care-of-it attitude (alas, not an uncommon one in some so-called "spiritual" circles) can give hope and faith a bad reputation.

To what degree do we create our own reality? Did we, in some way, choose this life, this family, these circumstances, these particular joys and troubles? If we could say for sure, we probably wouldn't need to be here anymore. But here we are. And if we conduct ourselves on the *presumption* that we participate in the creation of our reality, we avoid the anxiety that comes from perceiving ourselves as hapless victims.

*T*he more one sees life's connections and synchronicities, and even entertains the idea that one is playing a role in them, the more confident and the calmer one becomes. The calmer one becomes, the more connections are evident, and the more empowered one feels. It's a fine equation. And one that doesn't require too much scrutiny.

Accept it. Accept what life's mysterious maintaining forces give you. And give back to life what you can—with a Calm Mind at your service.

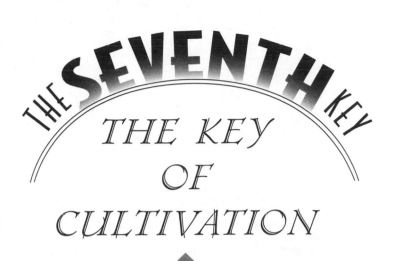

THE SEVENTH KEY

THE KEY
OF
CULTIVATION

◆

USE THE KEYS EVERY
DAY—ESPECIALLY WHEN YOU
LEAST FEEL LIKE IT.

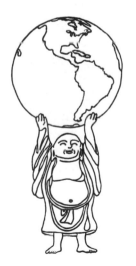

There was a student who was bothered by a spider every time he tried to quiet his mind. His master said, "Next time it happens, grab a brush and paint a circle on the spider's belly." The student did, and when he withdrew from his concentration he saw a circle painted on his own stomach.

—ZEN PARABLE

THE SEVENTH KEY TO CALM

Some of you have probably been following along with this book in an active fashion, incorporating the first Six Keys to Calm into your daily regime. Others of you may have decided to plunge ahead with reading, delaying your personal experience with the keys until you know exactly what it is you're "getting into" here. At this point, though, I'd like to suggest that those of you in the second group defer the reading of this final chapter until you have spent a few weeks practicing Keys One through Six.

To recap briefly, the use of the first Six Keys to Calm will take the following forms:

In keeping with the First Key, the Key of Clarity (which says *Be aware of what anxiety is and what it is not*), some ten minutes or so each day are dedicated to concentrating fully on a single, commonplace activity. The purpose of this is to begin to tame the Busy Mind, so it is not so easily distracted by "junk mail" thoughts that falsely signal apprehensive "red alerts."

In keeping with the Second Key, the Key of Compassion (which says *Substitute compassion for control*), motivations for helping those close to us are honestly examined. Also, each day a total stranger is assisted in a small, suitable way. These actions help us put aside anxious self-preoccupation, and also help us give up the illusion that we can control others.

In keeping with the Third Key, the Key of Crisis (which says *View each crisis as a crash course in calm*), our illusion that we can control the course of all events is challenged. The strength that all of us have found in times of gravest crisis is consciously recalled. And each day, a moment is taken to acknowledge a personal surrender to the flow of experience. In this way, we are able to take a break from our own exhausting defensiveness and appreciate how silly it is to imagine we can obliterate uncertainty.

In keeping with the Fourth Key, the Key of Cycles (which says *Celebrate change, because change is all there is*), we see that change and life are one and the same. Habitual anxious thought patterns that attempt to deny or defy change are countered by "looking for the strawberry," that is, by placing one's concentration on the most valuable element in any given situation. Now we are beginning to give up yet another anxiety-provoking illusion— the belief that we might stop time.

In keeping with the Fifth Key, the Key of Cessation (which says *Make an ally of your mortality*), new associations are made with regard to the concept of death. Rather than viewing it as a foe to be vanquished (which, of course, it can't), we view death as a counselor with worthy advice to offer. When we are anxiously torn between countless tasks and goals, we take mortality into account, asking, "Which of these things would I most like to be remembered for?" Now we can proceed with one positive aim in mind, calmly and completely.

In keeping with the Sixth Key, the Key of Connectedness (which says *Notice that life works*), we stay alert for signs that the universe is itself intelligent and compassionate. We collect evidence, by noting our own synchronous experiences and by looking around at the natural world. And we see that what looks, at first, like a jumbled-up mess often ends up making—quite literally—"perfect sense." By simply remaining observant, we realize that we probably have less to worry about than we imagined.

The Honeymoon Begins . . . and Ends

Now if you have been practicing the first Six Keys for even a few weeks, you have doubtless noticed that their cumulative effect has caused a number of things to happen. You are weaning yourself from ingrained habits. You are objectively observing your anxious impulses before acting on them. You are living more and more in the moment. You're not busy trying to "fix" everything all the time. And you're less obsessively attached to trivialities.

A new, increasingly composed outlook is becoming more and more your norm. In itself, this is quite an achievement. And yet, as you probably have also noticed, your calmness itself is engendering a number of beneficial side effects.

It's likely that you've noticed you are more observant, taking in your surroundings with a new level of interest and acuity. (I am always astonished how many people come into my office after embarking on the Seven Keys program and say things like, "What a lovely tree that is! A Norfolk pine, isn't it? When did you get it?" when, in fact, they'd passed it by for several months without a glance.) Liberated from continually worrying about what has happened or what might happen, you are naturally more perceptive and receptive to what's happening right now.

It's likely, too, that you've become more creative. No longer self-restricted to treading only familiar paths out of fear of the unanticipated, you are willing to experiment and enjoy the fruits of those experiments.

In the bargain, you have probably noticed improved relationships with others. This is because you have become both more approachable (no one gives "keep away" signals like an anxiety-ridden person, even if that's not what they consciously mean to convey) and less intimidating (now that you have given up trying to impose your agenda on people).

Finally, though it may seem strange, you may also experience yourself being more "lucky." Not lucky in the sense that you win a lottery jackpot, but in the sense that things generally seem to be going more smoothly than in the past, and that minor impediments no longer have the impact they once did. One might argue about whether such newfound "luck" is because those who trust the benevolent forces in the universe are most likely to benefit from them, or simply because to the calm person, what may have once seemed like a difficult circumstance now seems easily surmountable. I have come to believe it is a combination of both factors. But whatever the causes, it is a phenomenon numerous practitioners of the keys have reported.

With so many beneficial changes in the offing, what could possibly prevent one from using the Keys to Calm each and every day?

At first, not a thing. As a beginner you sail along, enjoying the perspective of the Calm Mind, and experiencing a redefinition of your very self. Where you once thought of yourself as intractably anxious, you now see yourself as fundamentally imperturbable. You contentedly think, "Hey, I wish I'd done this sooner," and "Now I'll do it forever."

But almost as soon as one thinks this, something else begins to take hold. The honeymoon—that sweet, initial period of full bedazzlement with something fresh and positive—appears to be on the wane. Perhaps a distraction of one sort or another (an important event, or a problem that demands attending to) looms large in your life. Suddenly, those few minutes and few actions a day you have devoted to stilling your Busy Mind seem like too much to spare, and the keys are abandoned with the well-meaning thought, "I'll get back to them soon." Or perhaps things have simply been going so smoothly that a sense of complacency sets in. Your practice of the keys seems to have been so effective that you think, "Well, I guess I don't need to do these so much—think I'll take a break."

Of course, before you know it, things seem to be backsliding to the way they were before. Those old, tenacious habits, so long in the making, have eagerly reaffixed themselves, like barnacles to the prow of your consciousness. You think of beginning to use the keys again but, unlike the first time you undertook their practice, you find yourself generating a significant amount of inertia.

There is a word for this self-generated psychic inertia. It is known as *resistance.* You may be most familiar with the term as it is used to describe, in electrical terms, the opposition of a body or substance to a current passing through it. In a way, it is used similarly here. The resistance of the Busy Mind to a new force attempting to pass through it is real—and considerable.

Psychic resistance is natural and inevitable. It makes sense that a reactive dragging of the heels occurs on the way to personal transformation. You have conducted yourself a certain way for your entire lifetime. To experience another way of being can be, in many ways, disconcerting. You may have had your complaints about your anxious habits but, after all, they were *familiar.* They went where you went, your faithful companions. In a sense you miss them, like you might long for an old, well-worn pair of shoes. Even if those shoes are long past practical usefulness, one may be wistful for them.

Still, the point of undertaking the Seven Keys program to begin with was to tap into a deeper, inner nature—a core of calm that lay dormant and undiscovered underneath familiar habits of the Busy Mind. Will resistance put an end to all your efforts? That *is* its agenda, but it need not prevail.

Resistance *can* be resolved, and that's what the Seventh Key is all about.

Understanding the Seventh Key to Calm

The Seventh Key to Calm says: *Use the keys every day—especially when you least feel like it.*

Absolutely everyone has days when, for one reason or another (and sometimes for no particular reason they can put their finger on), they are simply "not in the mood" to do the things that nurture them. On such days, vitamin pills go unswallowed, green vegetables go uneaten, and jogging shoes lie forlornly about, void of the feisty feet that only yesterday seemed so resolute. On such days, too, it is especially difficult to summon up the wherewithal to focus selectively on one activity, or to be alert to a stranger who requires assistance. One's attention is diffused; one's motivation dulled.

These are Resistance Days. Like double coupon days at the local supermarket, or alternate side of the street parking days in the city, they are regular occurrences. We will never be rid of Resistance Days. But we can decide what we are going to do about them.

In the past, when you committed a "sinful" omission—neglecting to eat your broccoli or trek over to the park for a morning run—you may have been excessively hard on yourself. You might have chastised yourself ("What a miserable lout I am!") and lamented that all your efforts so far were in vain ("I'll never really get anywhere").

Or, you may have been a bit too lax with yourself. You may have eagerly joined ranks with resistance, deluding yourself, day after day, into believing that you were only indulging in a brief hiatus from doing beneficial things. "I'll get back to it," you assure yourself, "whenever . . ."

As you may have noticed, neither of these reactions to your own resistance is particularly helpful.

The weight loss dieter who goes on a corn chip and nacho dip binge and mentally beats up on himself for it usually keeps eating, because he thinks "What's the use?" Likewise, the dieter who tells himself a few more chips (and a few more and more) won't really make a difference is also bound to perpetuate his own downward spiral.

The final part of the Seven Keys program is to make a conscious effort to avoid either of these paths. Doubtless you will have days when you ignore your Calm Mind, and forfeit being in the moment by dwelling on unsettling "what if" scenarios. Doubtless you will have days when you revert to wanting to "solve" everything—for yourself and everyone else. Having such days does not make you a bad person. On the other hand, letting one such day beget another and another is a sign that you are letting your Busy Mind trick you.

On Resistance Days, you can avoid the pitfalls of self-recrimination and of self-delusion. You can acknowledge that resistance is happening and you can persist in spite of it. You can do it by applying to resistance the salve of self-discipline.

The Key to Cultivation in Action

Now I can almost feel some of you cringing. *Self-discipline: What a drudge.* Perhaps when you think *discipline* you summon up visions of your childhood self sitting in the corner, enduring an embarrassing—not to mention boring—public penance. Or perhaps you conjure up an image of a completely spartan existence, one in which you will be required to shave your head, lose your shoes, don a modest robe, and subsist on bowls of brown rice. In the context of the Seven Keys program, however, neither of these scenarios is relevant. When it comes to cultivating calm, self-discipline is anything but constraining and limiting. It is, in fact, consummate liberation.

In the Seven Keys program, self-discipline is what will allow you to resolve resistance and to build up a *reservoir of calm* that will sustain you during your most stressful periods. Let me explain: Everyone tends to regress under stress. When the going gets rough, it is easy to "go into reverse" psychologically, undoing at least some of whatever progress one has recently made toward wearing in some new mental and emotional grooves. But the more faithful one is to maintaining one's progress each and every day, in good times and bad, without regard to external circumstances, the less intense that regression will be.

So, for example, if one has been practicing the Keys to Calm only "off and on" or "now and again" through a relatively stable time, and then runs across a major life disruption (a serious illness, for example, or relationship loss or financial reversal), one could easily lose ground to anxiety's powerful forces. If, however, that same person had been mindfully cultivating the Keys—even on Resistance Days—the scenario would alter. He might still slip backward a bit, at first, but instead of the dynamic being *two steps forward, two steps back,* it would be more like *two steps forward, a half-step back.* And because that same person would be able, ultimately, to learn even more about the inherent calm of his inner nature from any obstacle life put in his path, the overall picture would actually end up being *two steps forward, a half-step back, another step forward.*

So how, exactly, does one beat resistance? Well, you can't exactly beat it, and so you'll have to join it. In fact, the essence of self-discipline, in terms of the Seven Keys program, is to *outsmart resistance by using what it uses.*

Resistance is shameless. It will appropriate just about anything in your daily life to attempt to divert you from implementing the Keys to Calm. It will try to convince you that the endless chores and obligations of daily life are far too pressing to allow you to divert time and energy toward your practice. "How can you indulge in such extraneous undertakings," resistance will ask, "when you have memos to write, phone calls to return, meals to prepare, car pools to organize, laundry to sort, and homework to help with? You can't!"

Of course, if you look at the business of daily life as separate from your cultivation of calm, then you will have no choice but to give in to resistance and forgo your new habits. But the secret to resolving resistance is simply to remember this: *Carefully attending to the business of life and cultivating the Calm Mind are one and the same pursuit.*

Washing your clothes or assisting a child or working at your job with focused attentiveness, with positive intent, with compassion and sincerity, removes the anxious "either/or" factor from your thinking. Once you know this, you will never again need to worry about "choosing" whether to practice your keys or, say, get a casserole ready for dinner. You will no longer need to resent taking time away from *this* in order to do *that*. You will dice your vegetables and boil you noodles with care and mindfulness, and at the end of it all you will have a nice little supper and a composed perspective. And you will have knocked resistance for a loop.

Why did you want to access your Calm Mind in the first place? So you could "rise above" life, unfazed and uninvolved? Even if you could embody that attitude, you would hate it. (Not to mention the fact that you would also be wildly unpopular!) For you would stand apart from everyone and everything that gave existence meaning. No, the point of accessing the Calm Mind was—and is—so that you could embrace life in all its aspects, free of unwarranted fear, and diminish the distance that your nagging anxiety placed between you and your own immediate experience.

According to Zen Buddhist philosophy, even those who attain the summit of Enlightenment (the state of continually accessing one's Calm Mind) have achieved nothing special if they stay atop the mountain they have scaled. To realize and activate Enlightenment they must descend from the rarefied air and return to "the ten thousand things"—that is to say, to the joys and woes, the details and mundanities, the rituals and repetitions, the obstacles and challenges of down-and-dirty, in-your-face life.

This is your task as well. No matter how "high" or "above it all" the Seven Keys may make you feel from time to time, life is sure to reactivate your emotional gravity, bringing you down to earth again—sometimes with a humbling thud. And why shouldn't it? After all, there are places to go, people to see, things to do. So go to your places, see your people, and do the things you must. Just take your keys with you. They are infinitely portable. And unlike other keys, once you have them you can never really lose them. Even if you feel like you've misplaced them, you only need to look within to find them.

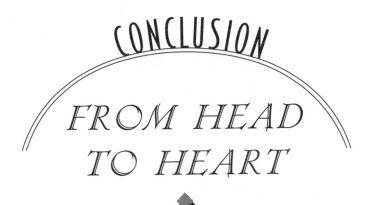

CONCLUSION

FROM HEAD TO HEART

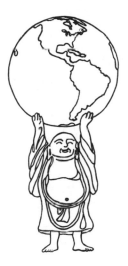

Whoever you are; some evening
    take a step
Out of your house, which you know
    so well.
Enormous space is near, your house lies
    where it begins . . .
                            —RAINER MARIA RILKE,
                                "The Way In"

When you come to a fork in the road,
take it.

                            —YOGI BERRA

At the start of this book, you were reminded of the story of the troll who became a prince, his transformation occurring ever so gradually from the outside-in. Keep in mind how different this story is from the run-of-the-mill fairy tale wherein changes occur instantaneously, via a wave of a magic wand or the whim of a transient gremlin.

It is a troll-into-prince sort of process that you should anticipate if you persist in using the *Seven*

Keys to Calm over time. Slow and subtle. Widening and deepening.

Never attempt to hurry it. And never imagine you are failing if at first you feel like you are walking about in someone else's shoes. Sooner or later, the shoes will fit.

Bit by bit, the things you first understood with your intellect will seep down into the core of your heart. When that happens, you may well realize that your newfound calm—even with all of its beneficial side effects—was not an end in itself, but the beginning of a new way of being in the world.

As the Calm Mind is accessed more and more, one's very perception alters. And when perception alters, experience necessarily alters as well.

For example, much of what we take to be the hard facts of our existence are not strictly facts at all. We see an object and name its color—a green leaf, an orange butterfly—but colors do not objectively exist outside of our own brains. There is no such "thing" as green or orange. There is only electromagnetic radiation, vibrating at a certain frequency. The same holds true for sound. You've doubtless heard the age-old philosophical question, If a tree falls in the forest and no one hears, does it make a sound? Actually, it does not. Sound itself is defined as the relationship between external vibrations and the brain.

Perception and what we call "reality" are co-influential. When the Calm Mind is doing the perceiving, one sees the world as a different sort of place. It is viewed as less threatening and more hospitable, less chaotic and more meaningful. As a result of revised perception, one responds differently to that world. One becomes less defensive and more attuned, less self-absorbed and more contributory. And most wondrous of all, as a result of that different response, the world, in some small but significant ways, actually becomes a different sort of place—not just to the original "perceiver" but to those who interact with him.

It is interesting indeed to envision a world where the force of the Calm Mind has become increasingly accessible to increasing numbers of people—a place where people examine their impulses before acting on them, for instance, and where they are committed to assisting one another in unobtrusive ways. One can only imagine how enhanced such a world might be. And one may even be tempted to try to figure out a way to *make it all come about* and *to bring everyone around as quickly as possible.*

But here I offer a final word of caution. The desire to "fix it all up" is your Busy Mind talking again. Though using the Keys to Calm may benefit you, do not take it upon yourself to foist a change upon anyone else who does not sense an internal readiness or manifest a significant curiosity.

People need to discover emotional truths for themselves, or else they won't feel true at all. As a therapist, and a parent, I am continually reminded of this dynamic (and should I temporarily ignore it, someone usually does me the favor of reminding me to get off my high horse).

You may be tempted to proselytize, to convert, to "solve" things for your friends and loved ones by pestering them into using the Seven Keys. Of course, people around you may notice the changes in you and may ask how and why they came about. Of course, you can discuss your experience to some extent (though part of it you'll find hard to describe in words). Of course, you can pass along a copy of this book (which itself is merely a catalyst for change). And of course, you can offer others support and wish them luck. But you cannot change them, only influence them. And the most effective way to influence people is simply to do what you have chosen to do, and do it to the best of your ability.

So go and do what you are going to do. And be who you have found out you really are. Be a living example—but without becoming a bore, if you please.

And the very best of luck to you.

NOTES ON SOURCES

Introduction

Alan Watts's quote is from his book *The Wisdom of Insecurity* (New York: Pantheon, 1951), p. 92.

The Hindu scripture quote is from *The Upanishads,* translated by Swami Prabhavananda and Frederick Manchester (Hollywood, Calif.: Vedanta Press, 1975), p. 177.

The First Key

The first epigraph is paraphrased from Watts, op. cit., p. 90.

The second epigraph is from the essay "Fancy Goods" in the German philosopher Walter Benjamin's *One Way Street* (1928).

Henry Miller's quote on awareness originally appeared in "Creative Death" in Miller's book, *The Wisdom of the Heart* (1947).

Krishnamurti's quote is from the essay "Can Thinking Solve Our Problems?" in *The First and Last Freedom* (New York: Harper & Row, 1954), p. 114.

The Second Key

The first epigraph is from Jack Kornfield's *A Path with Heart* (New York: Bantam, 1993), p. 217.

The second epigraph is from Chogyam Trungpa's *Cutting Through Spiritual Materialism* (Boulder, Colo.: Shambhala, 1973), p. 174.

Allan Sandage's comments on human origins are in Dennis Overbye's *Lonely Hearts of the Cosmos* (New York: HarperCollins, 1991), pp. 42–43.

The quote from Albert Einstein is from his *Ideas and Opinions,* translated by Sonja Bargmann (New York: Crown, 1954), quoted in *The Tibetan Book of Living and Dying,* by Sogyal Rinpoche (San Francisco: Harper San Francisco paperback edition, 1994), p. 98.

The lab experiment with cats was conducted by Paul Leyhausen and was cited in *When Elephants Weep,* by Jeffrey Moussaief Masson (New York: Delacorte: 1995), p. 56.

William Blake's quote is from *Jerusalem,* Ch. 3, Pl. 55 (in *Complete Writings,* 1804–20, edited by Geoffrey Keynes).

Freud's quote is from a footnote in *The Interpretation of Dreams,* Ch. 6, sec. E (1900, footnoted added in 1909), in Vol. 5 of *The Complete Works,* edited by James Strachey.

Carl Jung's quote is from *Psychology and Alchemy* (1944), in *Collected Works,* Vol. 12, edited by William McGuire.

Lewis Thomas's quote is from *The Medusa and the Snail* (New York: Viking, 1979), p. 106.

The quote on "friendliness to everything" is from Chogyam Trungpa, op. cit., p. 19.

The Third Key

The first epigraph is from Peter Matthiessen's *The Snow Leopard* (New York: Viking, 1978).

The second is from Krishnamurti's essay "On Simplicity," in *The First and Last Freedom,* op. cit., p. 272.

The third is from Richard Nixon's *Six Crises* (1962).

David Livingstone's memoir is cited in Lewis Thomas's *Lives of a Cell* (New York: Viking, 1974), p. 58.

The Tennessee Williams line is spoken by Chris in *The Milk Train Doesn't Stop Here Anymore* (1963), sc. 6.

Eugène Ionesco's quote is from "Have I Written Anti-Theatre?" in *Notes and Counter-Notes* (1962).

Watts's quote is from *The Wisdom of Insecurity,* op. cit., p. 94.

A story on the couple with the famed prenuptial agreement appeared in *Newsday,* on the front page of Pt. II (Feb. 1, 1996).

Henry Kissinger's quote is from *The New York Times Magazine* (June 1, 1969).

Richard Nixon's quote is from the introduction to *Six Crises,* op. cit.

Ryszard Kapuscinski's quote is from "A Warsaw Diary" (published in *Granta,* No. 15, Cambridge, England, 1985).

The Fourth Key

Freud's quote is from "Civilization and Its Discontents," in Vol. 21 of *The Complete Works.*

The Zen parable is recounted in *Zen Speaks: Shouts of Nothingness,* by Tsai Chih Chung, translated by Brian Bruya (New York: Anchor Books, 1994), p. 56.

Cézanne's quote is cited in *The Little Zen Companion,* by David Schiller (New York: Workman, 1994), p. 286.

The Fifth Key

The epigraph by Montaigne is from *The Essays of Michel de Montaigne,* translated and edited by M. A. Screech (London: Allen Lane, 1991), p. 95.

Shakespeare wrote of "the undiscovered country" in *Hamlet,* Act III, Sc. 1.

Timothy Leary was quoted in *The New York Times,* Nov. 26, 1995, and June 1, 1996.

The lines from Thornton Wilder's *Our Town* were spoken in Act III.

The story of Achaan Chaa and the broken glass is recounted in Mark Epstein's *Thoughts Without a Thinker* (New York: Basic Books, 1995), pp. 79–81.

The two Zen parables are from *Zen Speaks: Shouts of Nothingness,* op. cit., pp. 71 and 49, respectively.

The Buddha's comment on good deeds was found in *Buddha's Little Instruction Book,* by Jack Kornfield (New York: Bantam, 1994), p. 89.

Henry Ford's quote appeared in *Exploring Reincarnation,* by Hanns TenDam (London: Arkana, 1990), p. 377.

Voltaire's quote is cited in *The Tibetan Book of Living and Dying,* op. cit., p. 83.

Candace Pert's quote is from "Neuropeptides, the Emotions and Bodymind," in *Proceedings of the Symposium on Consciousness and Survival,* edited by John S. Spong (Sausalito, Calif.: Institute of Noetic Sciences, 1987), pp. 113–114.

Woody Allen's quote is from his essay collection, *Without Feathers* (1976).

Ivan Illich's quote appeared in *The Sunday Times* (London, Nov. 20, 1988).

The Sixth Key

The epigraph from Picasso was quoted in Jean Cocteau's *Opium* (1929), p. 29.

The epigraph by George Johnson is from his book, *Fire in the Mind* (New York: Alfred A. Knopf, 1995), p. 40.

Jung's quote on chaos is from "Archetypes of the Collective Unconscious," in Vol. 9 of *The Collected Works.*

David Bohm's theories are beautifully explained in *The Holographic Universe,* by Michael Talbot (New York: HarperCollins, 1991), pp. 32–55.

David Peat's book is *Synchronicity: The Bridge Between Mind and Matter* (New York: Bantam, 1987).

Lewis Thomas's quote is from an essay called "The Wonderful Mistake," in *The Medusa and the Snail,* op. cit., pp. 28–29 (the italics, however, were added by this author).

The story of the Buddha and the arrow is told in Lucien Stryk's *The World of the Buddha* (New York: Grove, Weidenfeld, 1968), pp. 52–53.

The Seventh Key

The Zen parable that serves as an epigraph to this chapter is from *Zen Speaks: Shouts of Nothingness,* op. cit., p. 69.

Conclusion

Yogi Berra's quote is from his commencement address at Montclair University, May 16, 1996 (though he undoubtedly said it before).

The interactions of color and sound with the brain were discussed by New York University neuroscientist Dr. Rodolfo Llinás, as quoted in *Time* (July 17, 1995), p. 52.